Chaga

Also by David Wolfe

Books

The Sunfood Diet Success System

Eating for Beauty

Naked Chocolate

Amazing Grace

Superfoods: The Food and Medicine of the Future

Longevity Now

DVDs

Superfood Recipes

Superherb Recipes

LongevityNOW Recipes

A Woman's Guide to Vibrant Health (Recipes)

Restoring Adrenal Health (Recipes)

Mega-Immunity (Recipes)

Affiliated Websites

www.davidwolfe.com

www.longevitywarehouse.com

www.thebestdayever.com

www.rawnutritioncertification.com

www.sacredchocolate.com

www.ftpf.org

Chaga

King of the
Medicinal Mushrooms

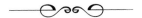

DAVID WOLFE

North Atlantic Books
Berkeley, California

Unless otherwise noted, all photographs were taken by David Wolfe (www.davidwolfe.com).

Special thanks to Andrea McGinnis for assistance on the beta glucans and chaga recipes sections, to Adam Collins of SuperfoodSnacks.com for his recipe additions, and to Frank Giglio for his recipe addition.

Published by
North Atlantic Books
Berkeley, California

Front-cover photograph of David Wolfe by Michael Roud. All other front-cover photographs by David Wolfe
Cover and book design by Brad Greene

Printed in the United States of America

Chaga: King of the Medicinal Mushrooms is sponsored and published by the Society for the Study of Native Arts and Sciences (dba North Atlantic Books), an educational nonprofit based in Berkeley, California, that collaborates with partners to develop cross-cultural perspectives, nurture holistic views of art, science, the humanities, and healing, and seed personal and global transformation by publishing work on the relationship of body, spirit, and nature.

North Atlantic Books' publications are available through most bookstores. For further information, visit our website at www.northatlanticbooks.com or call 800-733-3000.

MEDICAL DISCLAIMER: The following information is intended for general information purposes only. Individuals should always see their health care provider before administering any suggestions made in this book. Any application of the material set forth in the following pages is at the reader's discretion and is his or her sole responsibility.

Library of Congress Cataloging-in-Publication Data

Wolfe, David.
Chaga : king of the medicinal mushrooms / David Wolfe.
    p. cm.
  Includes bibliographical references and index.
  ISBN 978-1-58394-499-8
1. Mushrooms—Therapeutic use. 2. Medicinal plants. 3. Birch—Therapeutic use. I. Title.
  RM666.M87W65 2012
  615.3'21—dc23
                                                        2012012350

4 5 6 7 8 9 VERSA 20 19 18 17

North Atlantic Books is committed to the protection of our environment. We partner with FSC-certified printers using soy-based inks and print on recycled paper whenever possible.

This book is dedicated
to every wild mushroom hunter.

Mushroom hunting is
one of the greatest hobbies ever!

Acknowledgments

Cem Akin

Pierre Beaumier

Truth Calkins

Groovinda Dasi

Nathaniel Finkelstein

Len Foley

Scott Frasier

Juliana Garske

Lucien Gauthier

Rebecca Gauthier

Camille Perrin Giglio

Frank Giglio

Kathy Glass

Kohta Mitamura

Alan Muskat

Doug Reil

Krystyna Robin McMillan

Candice Richardson

Ramiz Saad

Thomas "Dandelion Hemp" Stinson

Wendy Taylor

Ron Teeguarden

Robert Weismandel

Contents

∾੭੬∾

Part I
Facts and History of Use . . . 13

❦

Part II
Preparing and Enjoying Chaga . . . 63

❦

Recipes ... 82

౬ఞఎ

Poetic Interlude
"Chaga, Philosopher-King" . . . 113

౬ఞఎ

Part III
The Science on Chaga . . . 121

౬ఞఎ

Part IV
Resources ... 155

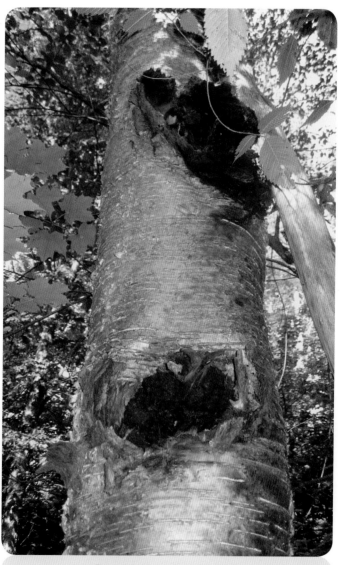

Superherb chaga

An Introduction to Superherbs

"Let food be thy medicine
and medicine be thy food."

—Hippocrates

This famous dictum—from a founder of Western medicine who championed treating the body as a whole and not just treating its parts—is frequently referenced and observed, cited and reflected upon, *but in only half its glory*. The first phrase, "Let food be thy medicine," is well known and understood by many, yet the second half of this age-old prescription contains what I perceive as the greater insight for our times. Eating medicine as food appears to be a literal statement. If we read Hippocrates literally, he is clearly telling us: eat herbal medicines regularly as food.

For thousands of years, the Shaolin monks (famous Buddhist warriors) and the Daoists of China gathered a wealth of information, wisdom, and knowledge about the medicinal properties of herbs, mushrooms, and other plants. And though they found many herbs wonderful as occasional foods, these same herbs were often inappropriate for consistent, daily use as food. However, the ancient Shaolin community recognized a distinction whereby the superior, "tonic" herbs were different and *could* be eaten regularly as food. A tonic is "tonifying," meaning that it is an overall health and wellness booster that helps restore, tone, and enliven body systems.

From my research, I find that the most powerful of these tonic herbs are the medicinal mushrooms (of which chaga is one), and they fall into a class I call "superherbs." Due to their naturally high nutritional and medicinal content, proven history, and whole-herb synergy, these superherbs have real potential for healing and invigorating us. I'm talking about more than sprinkling dried oregano on spaghetti. We can gain exponentially greater benefit from superherbs when we know how to incorporate them into our diet on a regular basis.

Over the last decade the Internet has become saturated with information on natural healing technologies, organic foods, raw foods, wild foods, herbal medicines, adaptogens, and especially the superherbs. Plant-based approaches to health challenges are increasing in popularity at an astonishing rate, probably because they work. We are nearing a critical mass of folks who are shifting their energy and financial power away from a bankrupt, misdirected, environmentally destructive pharmaceutical model of "disease care" to a sustainable, preventative, health-building, self-responsible model of wellness. Superherbs are likely our best allies in this global healing movement.

Following Hippocrates's dictum in its entirety to me implies exploring these tonic superherbs. And again, based on scientific research and the history of human usage, medicinal mushrooms crown the category.

It seems fitting to inaugurate a new series of books focused on the superherbs of our planet with chaga, fabled "king of the mushrooms," the bounds of whose beneficence have not yet been found.

David Wolfe's Top 25 Superherbs

NORTH AMERICA/EUROPE/RUSSIA/ASIA

Chaga—King of the medicinal mushrooms.

Horsetail—Ancient antifungal, Ormus-rich, bone-strengthening superherb.

Nettles—Anti-inflammatory, bone-building, blood-nourishing, testosterone-building, silica-gifting superherb: leaves and root.

Reishi—The most well-studied herb in the history of the world.

Rhodiola (Arctic root)—Adapt to less oxygen and improve your performance with this fitness super root.

CHINA

Ant—King of Herbs? No, Herb of Kings.

Astragalus—Nitrogen-fixing, temperate-climate super root that heals you with its polysaccharides and helps you live long with its astragalosides.

Deer Antler—Nature's source of hormone-building nutrients.

Ginseng—Even though its legend is as old as the hills, ginseng is still there to help heal you. Ginseng's magic will be with us forever. Use it.

Gynostemma—The longevity and health-building surprise of Chinese medicine.

Ho Shou Wu *(Polygonum multiflorum)*—Yin *jing*, bone marrow–nourishing, stem cell–building tonic, longevity, super root.

Schizandra Berry—This liver healer and antiviral is one of the most potent balancing herbs in Chinese medicine.

AMAZONIA AND THE ANDES

Cat's Claw—Invasive jungle plant that invasively protects your body from viruses and certain fungi.

Chanca Piedra—The "stone breaker" helps remove calcification in the kidneys, liver, and blood.

Coca Leaf—The most powerful food-herb on Earth; that's why it's illegal.

Pau d'Arco—Antifungal, anticandida, delicious super tea.

Sacha Jergon—Center of the Amazonian herbal-system medicine wheel.

CENTRAL AMERICA

Cayenne—This common herb packs some healing heat for cardiovascular problems.

Mucuna—Neurotransmitter-building, Parkinson's-fighting, super *jing* bean.

Vanilla—The world's greatest spice has medicinal properties.

INDIA

Ashwagandha—Adaptogenic, anthropomorphic super root.

Asparagus Root *(shatavari)*—Supertonic, longevity, fitness-improving properties are associated with this common garden plant and wild food found all over the world.

Shilajit—Mineral-pitch, super-resin Himalayan tonic that nourishes and detoxifies.

Tulsi—Adaptogenic superherb of Ayurveda.

SOUTHEAST ASIA

Mangosteen Rind—Antiarthritic, heal-everything superherb.

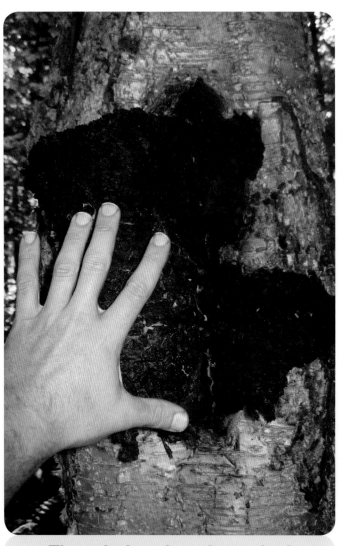

The relative size of a typical chaga specimen

Hail to the King!
An Introduction to Chaga

Chaga is a remarkable medicinal mushroom that grows in living trees. It grows most abundantly in nearly all species of birch found in the circumpolar temperate forests of Earth's northern hemisphere. As a food-herb and nutriment, chaga is a premier herbal adaptogen (a metabolic regulator that increases an organism's ability to adapt to environmental factors and resist stress), cancer fighter, immune-system modulator, antitumor agent, gastrointestinal (digestive) tonifier, longevity tonic, and a genoprotective (DNA-shielding) agent.

Latin Name

Inonotus obliquus

Regional Names

Clinker polypore, clinker fungus, cinder conk, tschaga (Russian), chaga (English adaptation of the Russian term), pakuri (Finnish), kreftkjuke (Norwegian), tschagapilz (German), kabanoanatake (Japanese)

A mainstay of traditional Siberian shamanism and healing, chaga has long been considered "king of the mushrooms." It continues to be highly regarded in Siberia (where chaga is used as a nutritional medicine and tonic) as an external treatment for the skin—in tea and wetted-poultice form, as an inhaled medicine (chaga smoke), and as a fire starter (kindling). Chaga is herbally recognized across Asia and is now rapidly gaining renown in Europe and North America.

Chaga is impressive in appearance and effect. You can tell people about its power and character, yet few can truly understand it until they experience it: the foamy, yellow-orange, dense chaga core; the scorched outer ridges; and the nutritionally rich, hardened layering found on the inner mushroom landscape in between.

In essence, chaga makes wood edible for humans. And what kind of wood? Primarily, it is the powerful medicinal wood of birch trees, chaga's preferred host. The rich tonics in birch bark are improved, concentrated, and delivered in an edible form by this superherb.

Chaga is part of the order of mushrooms known as Hymenochaetales, the members of which can affect dead wood and living trees. Like the highly acclaimed medicinal Polyporales (reishi, *Ganoderma* spp., *Fomitopsis* spp., *Grifola frondosa, Trametes versicolor,* etc.), some of the Hymenochaetales (notably chaga and *Phellinus* spp.) are considered to be members of a group of "medicinal mushrooms" because they have compounds

Superherb Type

TREE MUSHROOM

Chaga's Scientific Classification

Kingdom: Fungi
Subkingdom: Dikarya
Phylum: Basidiomycota
Subphylum: Agaricomycotina
Class: Agaricomycetes
Order: Hymenochaetales
Family: Hymenochaetaceae
Genus: Inonotus
Species: Obliquus

that positively influence the immune system, joints, and nervous system of mammals, including humans.

Medicinal mushrooms have super tonic and adaptogenic properties that allow you to consistently (even multiple times daily) ingest their nutrient-medicines that strengthen immunity; help fight allergies, asthma, and cancer; improve core vitality; and confer many other valuable gifts. For example, the fabled queen of the medicinal mushrooms, reishi *(Ganoderma lucidum),* helps support a healthy immune system, heart, lungs, and kidneys; lowers elevated blood pressure; and assists with rejuvenating brain and connective tissue—all while fighting allergies. As another example, the medicinal mushroom cordyceps *(Cordyceps sinensis)* fights fatigue, improves endurance, and increases both lung capacity and primordial life-force energy—what the Daoists call *jing* (which is a different energy from energy-flow *chi*, also spelled *qi*).

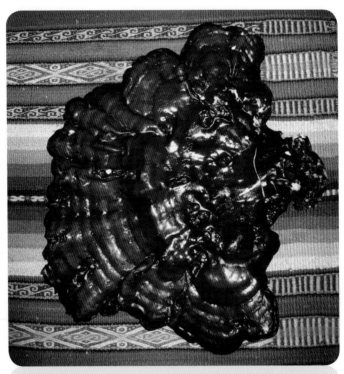

Reishi, Queen of the Medicinal Mushrooms, gains its brilliant red (sometimes purple or black) coloration from elongated hair-like cells (known as pilocystidia) embedded in a matrix of melanin pigments.

The king of the medicinal mushrooms, however, is chaga *(Inonotus obliquus)*—the subject of this book. This royal moniker comes down to us from traditional Siberian shamans, who crowned chaga the most powerful member of the mycelium kingdom. Chaga constitutes perhaps the greatest storehouse of medicinal healing properties of any single mushroom—or any herb, for that matter. In the following pages we will be exploring the extraordinary history, lore, research, and future of this potent healing mushroom.

Chaga's Unique Healing Powers

Diving right into it, we find that chaga's main distinction from other medicinal mushrooms is that it is composed of a dense configuration of antioxidant pigments. (Antioxidants and other constituents are discussed in depth in Part III.) Like other superherbs (e.g., *Astragalus membranaceus, Gynostemma pentaphyllum, Urtica dioica, Ganoderma lucidum,* et al.), chaga helps to reduce the workload of the immune system as a whole. Nearly every type of superherb has a different content of saponins and polysaccharides, with each combination helping to boost the activity of our immune cells in different ways. For example, each type of polysaccharide beta glucans molecule matches up with a specific type of cell in the immune system, each promoting a different immune response.

Various substances found in chaga possess powerful anticancer and antitumor properties. Many of chaga's anticancer properties are now being attributed to beta glucans and melanin, as well as to its other vitality- and longevity-inducing medicinal properties. Beta glucans are scientifically recognized as one

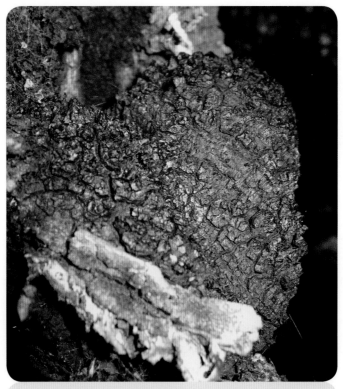

Chaga: King of the medicinal mushrooms

of the richest, most important forms of healing polysaccharides. Their discovery in the mycelium (netted, brainlike fungal structure) and in the fruiting bodies of medicinal mushrooms has led to major insights on the chemistry of how medicinal mushrooms work to heal the human body.

The efficacy of beta glucans is only one of the mechanisms by which chaga acts to resist cancer. In addition to beta glucans' polysaccharide superpowers that are explored in the pages ahead, chaga also contains notably high levels of the DNA-protective antioxidant known as melanin, which fights radiation and activates the pineal gland. Chaga's phytonutrients have an ability to inhibit nuclear factor kappa B—a compound known to cause healthy cells to mutate or self-destruct. The anticancer medicinal compounds betulin, betulinic acid, lupeol, and related triterpenes are also found in chaga. Anecdotal evidence from Russia associates consistent chaga intake with resistance to all cancers, all of which make chaga an excellent adjunctive superherb to support *any* cancer-fighting protocol.

The myriad benefits of this alkaline, medicinal tree mushroom can be gained in various forms. One can dry wild chaga and make teas with it; eat it fresh, or dry it and eat it; and make special alcohol and alchemical extracts from it. As this book reveals, there are many ways to bathe in its hidden powers!

Basically, there are benefits to every type of chaga product. We see this reflected across chaga literature and research worldwide. In a Russian atlas of medicinal plants, chaga is recommended as a tea, extract, or *nastoika* (tincture) for malignancies.[1] Dried wild chaga powder, simply eaten as food, appears to have healing effects on the digestive tract. In *MycoMedicinals, An Informational Treatise on Mushrooms,* fungal pioneer Paul Stamets summarizes the many unique uses for medicinal mushrooms in all possible forms (hot-water extraction, methanol, ethanol, and freeze-dried mycelium powder, etc.), all validated by scientific literature.[2]

The available information indicates that not only the tea, extract, and alcohol tincture of wild chaga have unique and valuable healing properties, but also that commercially available chaga mycelium powder (grown on a grain medium, not harvested in the wild) has great healing properties as well.

Chaga Safety

Chaga tea and chaga mycelium are safe and important health-food products for all ages (1 to 101+ years of age) and all stages of life, including pregnancy. Barring rare tree-mushroom allergies, pregnant women can take chaga tea and chaga mycelium daily during their entire pregnancy.

To date, no side effects or toxicity of chaga have been reported.

Luckily for all of us, chaga has already been classified by the United States Food and Drug Administration (FDA) as "food." Chaga has been granted GRAS status (Generally Recognized as Safe) from the World Health Organization. It is legal for distribution in the European Union, and it is classified as a medicinal mushroom by the World Trade Organization.

Denizen of an Enchanted Realm

The splendor of life forms that decorate this planet, including you, draw forth forces from inner enchanted realms that cannot be seen, heard, or otherwise easily detected. Behind the thin veil of the material world is an awe-inspiring universe of magic. Mushrooms emanate from this realm—and chaga is "king of the mushrooms." Consuming this legendary superherb helps us connect to that mysterious hidden world, brightening our day and activating our imagination. Chaga enhances the enchantment of being alive while delivering immediate benefits for healthy digestion, healing, nourishment, and longevity.

Chaga is a mysterious denizen of this Earth. It is one of the strangest creatures of the forest. Its burnt-charcoal, lightning-struck appearance is unmistakable.

Its properties—shocking. It seems that anybody who has studied the subject ultimately remains mystified by chaga.

Why does it do the reverse of every other mushroom? A typical tree mushroom grows its mycelium, or body, inside the tree, while chaga grows its "body," called a sclerotium, mostly outside the tree. (What most people

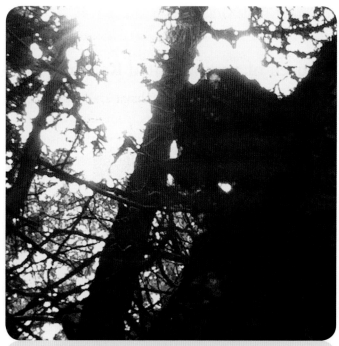

Chaga mushroom sclerotia interact with energies in the atmosphere.

visualize as mushrooms are actually the fruiting bodies—or reproductive organs—of various types of mycelium.)

As the chaga sclerotium grows, it slowly pushes the bark outward until it cracks it and eventually bursts forth from the trunk of the host tree (looking like a lateral or oblique frozen explosion of substance). With other types of tree mushrooms, you pick a soft or woody fruiting body on the outside of the tree. With chaga you pick the woody mycelium body or sclerotium. The only time a chaga will produce fruiting bodies is when its host tree dies. When the host tree dies, small brown-black chaga fruiting bodies (half-moon in shape) usually grow out of the chaga host tree near its base (or trunk).

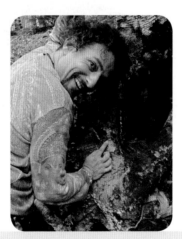

Chaga fruiting bodies—a rare phenomenon

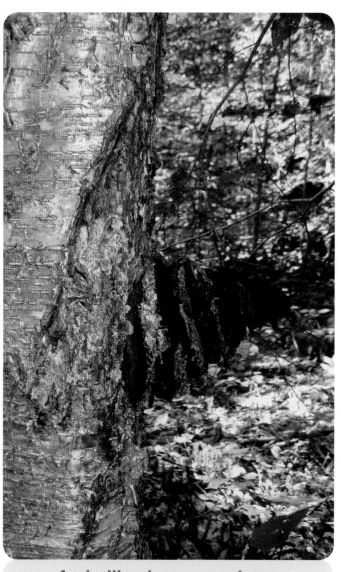

A phallic chaga specimen

Part I
Facts and History of Use

The medicinal mushroom known as chaga is harvested from living trees. Its "fruiting body"—called in English a sclerotium, or conk, or more technically, a herniated mycelium—emerges from the bark of chaga-bearing trees as a black, charcoal-like growth. The chaga conk is typically of irregular shape, although it is sometimes phallic. Upon removal of the chaga conk, a look at the interior of the mushroom reveals rusted-iron colors, twisted creamy veins, and layers of black-brown antioxidants. Its inner texture is similar to cork. In an article that became famous among chaga hunters, entitled "The Chaga Story" (published in *The Mycophile*), Ron Spinosa writes: "Some of those high-altitude [meaning high up in the tree] prizes may weigh over 10 pounds. The ideal chaga fruiting body is 25 years old."[1]

There are two primary methods employed by mushrooms to rot wood: brown rot and white rot. Wood is essentially composed of two classes of substances: cellulose (white matter), which is structural and forms the walls of plant cells, and lignins (brown matter), which form a second wall inside the primary cellulose wall. These lignins constitute 25% to 33% of the dry mass of wood. Brown-rot fungi degrade the white matter of cellulose, leaving the brown lignins behind. White-rot fungi break down dark lignins and leave white cellulose behind—hence the name "white rot."

Chaga is classified as a white-rot fungus in that it lives on the lignins in wood and therefore does not degrade the cellulose, which maintains the structural integrity of the living host tree. Actually, nearly all the medicinal tree mushrooms are white-rot fungi, including the following genera: *Ganoderma, Grifola, Phellinus, Polyporus,* and *Trametes.* This indicates that the primary food and mineral components of these medicinal mushrooms, including the levitative[2] hydrogen and Ormus elements, originate in the hydrophobic lignans or are drawn from the hydrophilic polysaccharides interwoven (in Fibonacci sequences) in the lignins of tree wood. I suspect that this is an important clue in developing future super-medicines from the medicinal mushrooms—it's an insight into how to give these healing substances more of the nutriment they want, so they become more potent.

Chaga in the Wild

A resident of temperate forests in the northern hemisphere, chaga prefers growing in living birch trees (genus: *Betula*) near springs, riparian areas of streams, wetlands, and marshy regions, though I have seen chaga growing on birch trees rooted in crevasses and rocky crags of hills and mountains. Chaga seems to favor yellow birch and white birch above all host trees. It may also grow in alder, ash, beech, elm, ironwood, and maple trees, albeit rarely, and occasionally in apple trees.

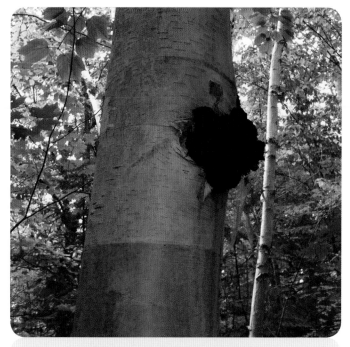

**Chaga concentrates
the medicines (such as betulin,
betulinic acid, and lupeol)
found in birch bark.**

Chaga loves the cold. As long as birch can grow, then the colder the weather, the better. Chaga is said to love −40°F (−40°C; they are the same temperature).

It is estimated that only about 0.025% of trees (that's only five for every 20,000 trees) will grow a chaga mushroom. I have found chaga to be slightly more common.[3] Nevertheless, the chaga mushroom is relatively rare, even in its prime growing regions.

Like reishi mushrooms, chaga seems to grow within trees that stand in very special places in the forest—usually on power spots. For example, we found a giant chaga while visiting the Temple of Lemminkäinen (one of the most sacred sites in Finland). Featured prominently in Ior Bock's saga of the Finnish people and their version of the creation of the world, this magical place was said to be a storehouse of unknown treasures, and its location was at one time the North Pole.

There are competing theories about the nature and life cycle of chaga. Some researchers argue that chaga is parasitic to birch, or that it is a "cancer of the birch tree" (as Russian novelist Aleksandr Solzhenitsyn wrote), causing its early demise in a cycle that takes about twenty years. Some say chaga takes down birch trees that are only five to seven years of age, which I definitely know is not true. I have seen chaga conks growing on birch trees that were closer to fifty years old and doing perfectly fine, and I have observed chaga growing on specific trees for seven-plus years.

There appears to be some evidence that chaga scle-rotia will erupt where birch trees have been injured or damaged. My experience indicates that this is not where the chaga mushroom gets into the tree, but it is where the chaga grows to protect the tree.

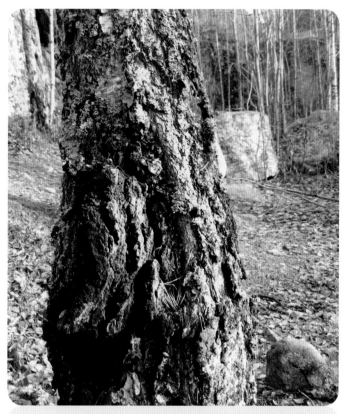

**Chaga growing at the Temple
of Lemminkäinen**

The alternative to the theory of chaga as parasite is the observation and belief that chaga grows in partnership with a living tree and has a symbiotic relationship with its host (this is the theory that I support). For this reason, chaga is called an endophytic mushroom, meaning that it can live within another plant symbiotically for part or all of its life without causing apparent disease.

The chaga and the birch take something they need from each other. In this model, chaga can even be seen as a protective force, because it improves the "immune system" of the host tree (as we have seen, that usually means a type of birch) and the forest itself. Research cited by Paul Stamets in *Mycelium Running* indicates that chaga extracts can be used topically against tree diseases (not just on birch trees), applied directly to the area of infection—further validating the symbiotic model of chaga. He details the story of a Quebec arborist who used chaga as a poultice to heal chestnut blight. Not only did this save the tree from its immediate crisis, but the tree's immune system was also permanently improved and became more resistant to future infections.[4]

In fact, chaga's theme—at one time a mystery of Nature but now slowly being revealed—is that it is healing. It heals plants, and it heals you by its phytochemistry (and by getting you up and into the woods to go look for it!).

Is Chaga an Extremophile?

Despite chaga's affinity for cold weather, it apparently can survive both heat and digestion. One could say it not only promotes longevity in those who consume it—chaga is itself extremely long-lived and hardy.

My neighbors noted that while they were consuming wild chaga (almost exclusively as boiled tea), mycelium spindles would be found in their composting toilet. These bundles became very hard over time and could not be processed the way they normally processed their "humanure."

This anecdotal report led to my own subsequent research that now indicates that some aspect of the chaga organism, even in tea form, somehow survives being heated—even boiled—and that the aspect of chaga that survives will grow into spindly, mycelium-like structures once returned to an earthy, wood decay environment.

This may indicate that chaga—like wild *Cordyceps sinensis* and lichen (a mushroom–algae symbiont)—consists of two or more organisms living symbiotically, one of them an extremophile (probably from the great living kingdom of *Archaea*) with extraordinary survival capabilities. If true, this discovery overturns the traditional scientific assumption that chaga sclerotia are sterile. More research is required in this area.

◄○►

The Birch Tree: A Most Excellent Host

Birch is by nature and essence an edible and medicinal tree. One can conclude from a summary of worldwide research on birch that no other tree can match the multiple medicinal uses of many of its components (bark, leaves, buds, sap, wood, and associated fungi: chaga, birch polypore, *Phellinus* spp., *Pholiota* spp., *Amanita muscaria/pantherina, Fomes fomentarius*). Birch is a staple of folk medicine, and its health benefits have been scientifically proven as well.

In Iceland, the endemic birch trees were almost completely eaten by introduced sheep (nearly eliminating birch in the wilds of that island), probably because of the exceptional taste and medicinal properties of birch that these animals are instinctively attracted to. Young, medicinally active birch trees stand no chance against hungry sheep.

Birch bark, in its own right, is a powerful medicine and is great in tea. Interestingly, birch bark tends to have a wintergreen flavor when made into tea; however, this flavor does not pass into the chaga. Medicinal wintergreen compounds in birch bark therefore appear to be of a different character entirely than the betulin, betulinic acid, lupeol, and other medicinal compounds found in chaga. These wintergreen compounds may (or may not) have something to do with the birch tree's special ability to purify the atmosphere. Scientists Tulchinskaya and Yurgelaytis report that in the atmosphere of a birch forest, there are 400 microbes per cubic meter, which is lower than the existing standards for hospital operating rooms.[5]

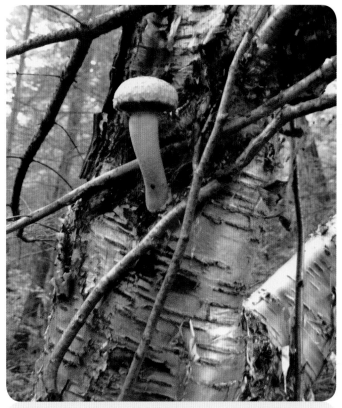

A *Pholiota* mushroom growing on birch

Birch was extensively utilized by the Native Americans of the northeastern United States and eastern Canada, not only as food, tea, and medicine, but also to create berry baskets and other containers and tools.

The Finnish and Russian people to this day, while heating themselves up in a sauna, take arm-length, fresh, birch branches with the leaves, wet them in spring water, heat them over the rocks, and then beat their bare skin with them for therapeutic effects.

Russian folklore implies that in the regions where birch bark is traditionally used in household articles such as baskets, boxes, hats, and food- and chaga-storage containers, people live longer and cancer rates are lower.

The *RigVeda,* a collection of ancient Indo-European poems, prayers and songs, is considered to be the earliest literary document in the world. A manuscript of the *RigVeda* from Kashmir, was found to be written on birch bark, in the *Sharada* script (pre-dating *Sanskrit*).

Burning birch in a stove never seems to leave any toxic fumes in the house. The birch bark also crackles when it starts burning, creating an exquisite sound.

Additionally, birch sap is the original and purest source of the impressive sweetener xylitol *(see page 83).*

Overall, birch trees appear to return health to the land. They pioneer disturbed sites. They act as nurse trees to nourish a damaged forest back to health via the following routes: endophytic symbiosis with tree mushrooms (enriching and encouraging mycelium in the soil); offering animals food; delivering medicinal compounds to animals of all types and even to the soil itself; purifying the atmosphere; and increasing the overall beauty of the forest.

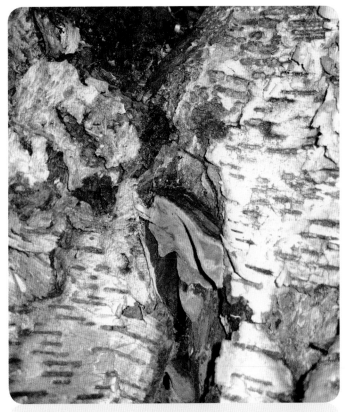

Chaga (above) growing with the polypore *Phellinus* (below)

Chaga: History, Literature, Legend

Just as ancient folk wisdom positions the lion as the king of the jungle, European, Finnish, and Russian lore positions chaga as the king of the temperate boreal forest. These native folk-medicine traditions ascribe unlimited benefits to chaga. Present-day scientific and medical research continues to validate the intuitive knowledge of these traditions, carefully adding even more benefits to an already long list.

In my introduction to chaga (pages 1–11), I touched on the well-established role of chaga in Siberia, where it has long been consumed as a medicine and a daily tea, inhaled as smoke, used as an external treatment for skin, and utilized as a form of kindling. Its ancient history of use extends across Asia from Europe to Japan.

The Chinese book *Shennong Ben Cao Jing* names chaga as a superior medicinal herb (according to Internet sources).[6] It is speculated that this agriculture and medicinal-plant book was written around 2800 BCE. The original text no longer exists but is said to have been composed of three volumes containing 365 entries on medicaments and their descriptions.[7] Chaga is known to nourish two Daoist tonic herbal treasures: *jing* (primordial energy) and *shen* (spiritual aura).

Undoubtedly, chaga was intertwined in the shamanic mix of events when the Santa Claus myth[8] arose in Northern Europe out of the shamanic, visionary, slightly toxic psychedelic mushroom *Amanita muscaria* (*Amanita pantherina* in America). From an archetypal perspective, *Amanita muscaria* is the joker or jester in the court—the fool, so to speak. It has many faces and a great deal of potential for toxicity but occasionally hits just right. Due to its uncertain aspects, *Amanita muscaria* has never been very popular. In the temperate forests of Canada where I hunt chaga, wild *Amanita pantherina* grows, and it seems to provide a more positive experience when dried upside down in direct sunlight and taken with chaga tea. I stumbled across this by studying the archetype: the king tells the jester what to do and keeps the jester in line.

It is unclear to me if and where chaga was utilized by North American native peoples. Cherokee descendants claim that chaga was known and used by their ancestors. Certainly many tribes of Algonquin peoples and the natives of Appalachia have been using birch bark as medicine for thousands of years, but information on their use of chaga is unsubstantiated in any literature I researched on the subject. Clearly more study is required.

I'd like to share a mytho-historical legend from Ireland here, the actual "truth" of which has slipped into the mists of time but a legend which nonetheless appears to have chaga's signature written all over it:

According to old Irish mythology, Tir Nanog is physically located at Mt. Brandon, Ireland, the western-most point of Eurasia, where the Irish Goddess Brigid lives in a sacred grove of twenty birch trees. To those who come to Her, she provides a divine herb (a special mushroom) that grows in Her sacred grove of birch trees.

Brigid's divine mushrooms confer healing and immortality on those who eat them by re-activating their Nanog gene. They then remain forever young, and are continually regenerated.[9]

Secrets of the Iceman

A relatively recent accidental discovery sheds an intriguing light on the widespread historical use of medicinal mushrooms. On September 19, 1991, two German tourists discovered the preserved remains of what became known as "Otzi the Iceman" in a melting glacier in the Austrian–Italian Alps. News of this find reached the world media. Subsequent scientific investigation indicated that Otzi lived approximately 5,100 to 5,350 years ago. He died (probably of an arrow wound) between the ages of forty and forty-five. Of particular interest was that three fungal objects were found amongst numerous items in the Iceman's equipment. The so-called "Black Matter" filling up the major part of the "girdle bag" was originally thought to be resin or chaga. The "Black Matter" was eventually shown to be a prepared tinder material that consisted of loose *hyphae* (dry filaments) made from the polypore *Fomes fomentarius*. The two objects on the leather thongs were identified as fruit body fragments of the polypore *Piptoporus betulinus* or Birch Polypore.[9a] Researchers believe that Otzi and his people used *F. fomentarius,* to start fires (as a portable form of kindling); and used both mushrooms to prevent bacterial and viral infections, heal wounds, and treat intestinal parasites.[9b] The portability, medicinal concentration, and multiple practical uses of medicinal mushrooms make them an obvious choice for ancient people. The iceman discovery clearly confirms what mushroom researchers have suspected for decades—that medicinal tree mushrooms have been utilized for an extraordinarily long span of human history.

Other Traditional and Practical Uses

Chaga Drums—According to my colleagues in Finland, in a past era large chaga sclerotia were cored and dried. A dried chaga like this would have the shape of a horn. A prepared animal skin was pulled over the hole to create a shaman's drum.

Clothing Dye—Chaga has been, and continues to be, used as a clothing dye. I personally use chaga for this purpose to capture some of its royal essence in my clothes. Simply boil wild chaga in a large pot of water for several hours. Wait until the chaga tea turns a deep scarlet color. Once the tea has cooled below the scalding level, add the clothing and soak it for 24 to 36 hours. Remove and wring out the clothing, then hang dry, preferably outside.

Fire Starter—Together with the tree mushroom *Fomes fomentarius*, dried chaga was used for thousands of years as tinder to help start fires with primitive flint-spark tools (e.g., the Iceman's supply). Traditionally, the yellow-orange core material of the chaga was dried, urinated upon, then dried again (this can be repeated numerous times)—a method of increasing the chaga's flammability. This is not unusual. Many Westerners have

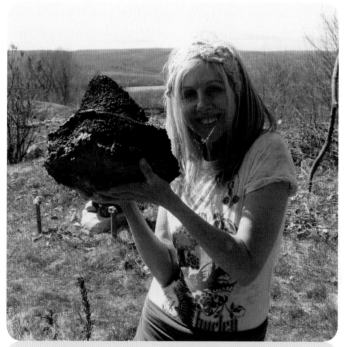

This type of chaga could be hollowed out to form a drum.

forgotten that gunpowder was originally made from processing human urine and feces.

In the colloquial language of those who teach survival skills, chaga is a "coal extender." Once prepared and lit, it is difficult to put out. The role of *Fomes fomentarius* was to provide dry tinder when busted apart by a rock, and this then could catch a spark, thereby complementing chaga in this early fire-starter

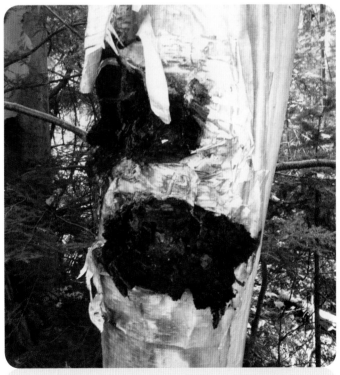

A birch tree stained by chaga

kit. Another method was to create a deep hole in the *Fomes fomentarius,* in which a piece of hot chaga coal could be placed. If the hole was properly burrowed and a suitable piece retained, the cap could be placed back over the hole, allowing one to travel with a live ember.

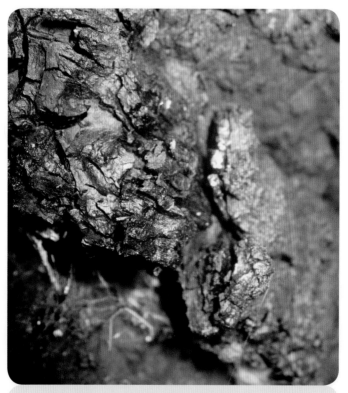

Chaga is a coal extender and has helped humanity utilize fire for millennia.

Chaga's Literary Debut

Chaga was most notably introduced to the West by Russian writer Aleksandr Solzhenitsyn's somewhat autobiographical novel *The Cancer Ward*. The book was initially published in the Soviet Union in 1968 and was immediately banned; its first English publication appeared in 1969. *The Cancer Ward* is the story of several cancer patients in the Soviet state of Uzbekistan in the year 1955. The novel explores themes of guilt, fear, moral responsibility, hope against impossible odds, and the metaphorical meaning of cancerous tumors, all in the shadow of Stalin's brutal regime. Solzhenitsyn is represented by his protagonist, Oleg Kostoglotov.

> They sighed. All of them, those who had left Central Russia long ago, some even voluntarily, as the ones who had never even been there, all now had a vision of that country, unassuming, temperate, unscorched by the sun, seen through a haze of thin sunlit rain, or in the spring floods with the muddy fields and forest roads, a quiet land where the simple forest tree is so useful and necessary to man. The people who live in those parts do not always appreciate their home; they yearn for bright blue seas and banana groves. But no, this is what man really needs: the hideous black growth on the bright birch tree, its sickness, its tumor. . . . Only Musalimov and Egenberdiev thought to themselves that

here too, in the plains and on the hills, there was bound to be just what they needed; because man is provided with all he needs in every corner of the Earth, he only has to know where to look.[10]

The following oft-quoted passage is famous in chaga lore, possibly because it hints of chaga's secret message:

Kostoglotov himself...had no one in Russia he could ask to look for the fungus. The people he knew were either already dead or scattered about the country, or he'd have felt awkward about approaching them; others were complete cityites who'd never be able to find the right birch tree, let alone the chaga on it. He could not imagine any greater joy than to go away into the woods for months on end, to break off this chaga, crumble it, boil it up on a campfire, drink it and get well like an animal. To walk through the forest for months, to know no other care than to get better! Just as a dog goes to search for some mysterious grass that will save him. But the way to Russia was forbidden to him.

As Solzhenitsyn describes, the ideal of chaga gives you the single-pointed focus to heal yourself, to wander the forest like a wounded animal after one goal: to get well. Having worked in the alternative-health field for twenty years, I find this to be profound.

More Polypore Lore, Geology Mythology, and Atmospheric Spores

There is a story circulating among mushroom researchers that I believe has validity and deserves its day in the Sun (pun intended). It gained popularity in certain circles due to the activism of magic-mushroom psychonaut, author, and lecturer Terence McKenna during

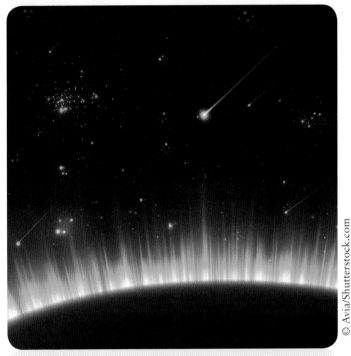

Cosmic mushroom spore dust

the latter half of his career, prior to his untimely death in 1999. I have spent quite some time meditating on this story and making natural observations that relate to it. Due to my experience as a wild mushroom hunter and researcher, I believe that I have been able to flesh out a bit more of the story and its significance.

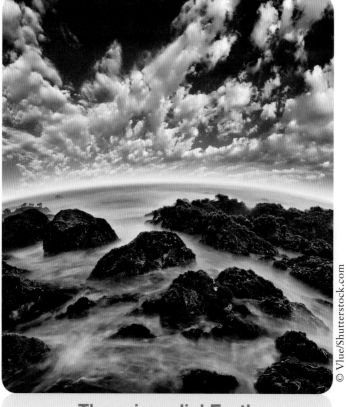

© Vlue/Shutterstock.com

The primordial Earth

According to legend, originally (perhaps millions or even billions of years ago), dormant mushroom spores from distant planets were carried by cosmic winds or meteors into the Earth's atmosphere. The spores subsequently deposited themselves upon the lands and waterways. As primitive bacterial and algae life forms developed, multiplied, and moved upon the land, their carbon and silicon wastes eventually formed a soil substrate that allowed the mushroom spores to leave their dormant state and "sprout" into mycelium-developing mushroom organisms whose preliminary evolutionary goal was to establish an ecosystem of multicelled organisms.

The preliminary work develops as the mushroom mycelium sets itself up to network and nourish multicelled carbohydrate-forming organisms (chlorophyll-gifted organisms). In return, the mushrooms are fed nutrients by these chlorophyll-rich plants.[11] Eventually, the way is paved for the roots of multicelled land shrubs and trees while helping to build soil, a process that eventually culminates in the development of lush forests.

In addition, the running mycelium in the soil protects local DNA from cosmic and volcanic radiation damage, sponges up radioactive isotopes, and detoxifies the environment.[12]

The ultimate evolutionary goal of the mushroom (in the cosmic vision) is to generate vast, inspired forestscapes, at which time an aspect of the mushroom kingdom evolves into polypores (wood-eating mushrooms like chaga). Wood is a more ennobled substrate or growth medium for mushrooms than a chaotic and mixed soil environment. The polypore works to liberate powerful levitational (upward-tending; see note 2) forces, monoatomic (Ormus) minerals (which are met-

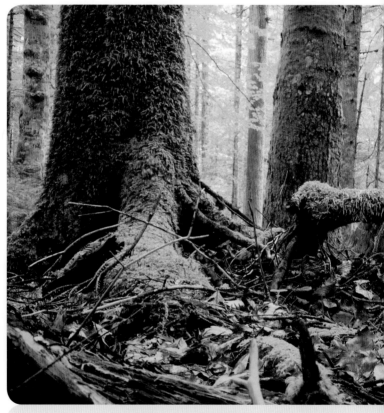

Mushrooms help transform

als that behave like ceramics), metals, sulfur, silicon, carbon, and hydrogen from the Earth and atmosphere. These elements and forces are concentrated by trees and reconcentrated by polypores in order to form fruiting bodies and spores. Because of each tree's affinity for levitational matter (in particular, hydrogen, sulfur, carbon,

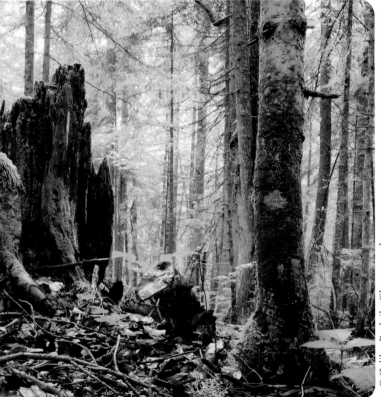

bare rock into lush forest.

© Zeljko Radojko/Shutterstock.com

and Ormus minerals), they concentrate these substances over their lifetime, eventually accumulating enough to create potent spores in fungal growth.

My observations have taught me that when a polypore mushroom releases its spores, they come out in a puff, as part of a highly energetic action, and levitate upward, like smoke. The spores are then borne upon the wind and carried both near and far.

Continuing the cosmic vision, a spore's eventual goal is to be carried back into space in its attempt to fall into the Sun. Levity on Earth basically means the inherent "desire" to fall into the Sun.

The polypore spores, upon dispersal, contain enough levitative substances (with inherent attraction to the Sun) and perfection in their geometries of shape (spherical and egg shapes) that, through the Coriolis action of weather and wind, they can be carried so high that some actually escape the Earth's atmosphere and enter into the vacuum of space on their way to the Sun. Through the slingshot effect, some of these spores could be hurtled to the outer planets and eventually out of the solar system. Others would fall into the Sun or simply be destroyed by cosmic forces.

The surviving spores travel with new information about planet Earth and upgraded genetics from their experience here. Eventually these spores may find a new home on another young planet, where the ecosystem-building process can begin anew.

The "raw Earth to forestscape" developmental processes may take millions or billions of years. In the meantime, the mushrooms develop themselves and other life forms by helping to construct healthier soil life and plants, building the foundation for trees and forests (as we have seen) and, importantly, acting as medicines for conscious beings that develop on that

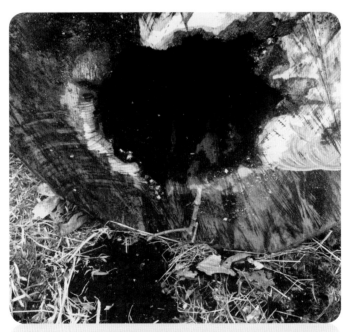

Trees concentrate within themselves ennobled growth materials and even "soils" that mushrooms eat to produce levitational spores.

planet with powers to significantly modify their environments and nutriment (in our case: humans).

Research indicates that mushroom spores are electron-dense and can survive the vacuum of space.[13] My review of the information on spores indicates that the outer material of the mushroom spore appears to be metallic in nature, and just beneath that metal shielding are layers of light monoatomic (Ormus) elements that shield the genetic material from radiation and possess levitative properties, such as an attraction to the Sun.

According to Terence McKenna:

> Global currents may form on the outside of the spore. The spores are very light and by Brownian motion are capable of percolation to the edge of the planet's atmosphere. Then, through interaction with energetic particles, some small number could actually escape into space. Understand that this is an evolutionary strategy where only one in many billions of spores actually makes the transition between the stars—a biological strategy for radiating throughout the galaxy without a technology. Of course this happens over very long periods of time. But if you think that the galaxy is roughly 100,000 light-years from edge to edge, if something were moving only one one-hundredth the speed of light—now that's not a tremendous speed that presents problems to any advanced technology— it could cross the galaxy in one hundred million

years. There's life on this planet 1.8 billion years old; that's eighteen times longer than one hundred million years. So, looking at the galaxy on those time scales, one sees that the percolation of spores between the stars is a perfectly viable strategy for biology. It might take millions of years, but it's the same principle by which plants migrate into a desert or across an ocean.[14]

This idea that mushrooms can be introduced to the Earth's environment from extraterrestrial sources has cultural and historical precedent. A disintegrating meteor that penetrates the Earth's troposphere may discharge enough particulate matter to generate the nuclei for cloud condensation, resulting in clouds that eventually pour spore-filled rain onto the ground.[15]

Going a bit further, the general idea that life filtered into the Earth environment from the cosmos is gaining scientific credibility. Francis Crick, who with James Watson discovered the structure of DNA, wrote a book on the cosmic origins of the genetic code.[16] He called this theory "directed panspermia." His argument was based on the concept that it is mathematically impossible for the genetic code to have randomly arisen in the early history of the Earth. During the 1960s, two British astronomers, Sir Fred Hoyle and Dr. Nalin Chandra Wickramasinghe, researched the nature of galactic dust. They concluded that this dust consists mostly of freeze-dried bacteria.[17]

Charles Fort, in his famous contrarian work *The Book of the Damned*, cites hundreds of well-documented historical cases of strange objects falling from the sky, including red, black, and yellow rains, thunderstones, chunks of earth, cinders, coal, bizarre giant hail, worms,

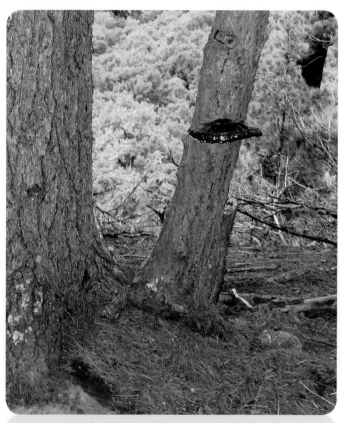

Are mushrooms from outer space? You decide.

frogs, fish, and other items that completely violate our current theory of reality and cannot be accounted for by the usual excuse of whirlwinds or tornados. Many of the rains brought mushroom species to the Earth that were later identified as "nostoc," a term that once referred to gelatinous mushroom material and is now identified with cyanobacteria. Fort argued that, according to clear evidence, the mushrooms were brought down from the heavens; whereas his religiously scientific contemporaries claimed that the mushrooms must have been here on Earth "in the first place" even though the actual evidence has never supported this.

Different types of mushroom spores (such as wheat rust) are known to travel great distances and to attain high altitudes.

In the early days of the age of aviation, a new science was born—aerobiology. During the 1930s, mushroom spore samples were obtained at altitudes of 3,000+ meters. Charles Lindbergh, in collaboration with the United States Department of Agriculture, participated in surveying spores while he was flying over the Arctic Circle. At altitudes of 1,000 meters, Lindbergh was able to catch what was described as a "considerable number of spores" far from land, over open ocean.

Later, more sophisticated experiments utilized balloons to find spores at higher elevations. In 1935, the balloon *Explorer II* was released at an altitude of 71,395 feet. It contained a spore-trapping device that was set to close once the balloon dropped to 36,000 feet. Five living spores were recovered. At the elevations in which the spores were trapped, winds were measured at 40 to 60 miles per hour, and temperatures were below freezing. If winds remained constant at those elevations, it was calculated that fungal spores up in this jet stream could be carried 8,400 miles in a week.[18] It appears there is an entire atmospheric ecosystem that is just coming to light.[19]

Chaga's Nutrients

Chaga's amazing nutritional profile continues to be uncovered by research. This section provides a summary of the important constituents of this powerful superherb, while Part III offers more scientific details and references for those who want additional information.

Antioxidants

Chaga is composed of a notably dense configuration of antioxidant pigments. In research sponsored by me and performed by Brunswick Labs (dated March 11, 2011), raw, dried, wild American chaga tested at 282 micromoles TE per gram; 247 micromoles TE per gram of this ORAC score (oxygen radical absorbance capacity, a measure of antioxidant content) turned out to be water-soluble. Interestingly, only 35 micromoles TE per gram were fat-, oil-, and lipid-soluble. This indicates that most of chaga's antioxidants will be extracted in hot water.[20]

Chaga is one of the best natural sources of the super-antioxidant, liver-cleansing, cell membrane–protective, genoprotective, longevity enzyme known as superoxide dismutase (SOD). Chaga contains more SOD than other rich sources such as barleygrass, seaweeds, marine oils, and even some essential oils. Chaga contains 25 to 50 times more SOD than other medicinal mushrooms

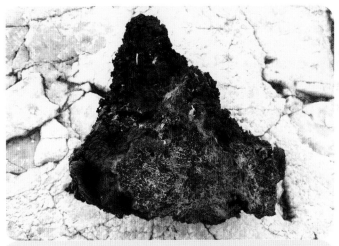

Chaga's rich blacks, browns, and oranges are derived from its high-molecular-weight, dark melanin pigments crossed with its low-molecular-weight, styrylpyrone-class phenol yellow pigments. These pigments demonstrate powerful antioxidant, anti-inflammatory, anti-platelet aggregation, anti-diabetic, anti-tumor, and anti-viral effects.[20a]

(reishi, maitake, shiitake, etc.).[21] In volumetric (liter-based) research sponsored by the Dove Health Alliance and performed by Brunswick Labs (dated September 27, 2005), wild Siberian chaga alcohol tincture tested at 3,781 kilo-units SOD-equivalent per liter. This is an exceptionally high reading. By volumetric comparison to other medicinal mushrooms, maitake tested at 85, cordyceps at 81, reishi at 23, and agaricus at 24 (k-unit SOD-eq per liter).

By mass (gram-based) comparison, mushroom SOD concentrations were detected as follows (in units per gram):

Truffles	860
Reishi	1,400
Agaricus	1,500
Siberian chaga	35,000[22]

Vitamins, Minerals, and Other Nutrients

Data from research conducted at facilities all over the world indicate that chaga contains not only an extraordinary level of antioxidants, but also a full assortment of healing nutrients, including polysaccharides (beta glucans, protein-bound xylogalactoglucans, etc.), polyphenols, sterols (lanosterols/ergosterols), inotodiols, triterpenoidal saponins, melanin, betulin/betulinic acid, lupeol, trace minerals (antimony, barium, bismuth, boron, chromium, copper, germanium, manganese, selenium, zinc), major minerals (calcium, cesium, iron, magnesium, phosphorus, potassium, rubidium, silicon, sulfur), vitamins (B_2, D_2), dietary fiber, and amino acid complexes.

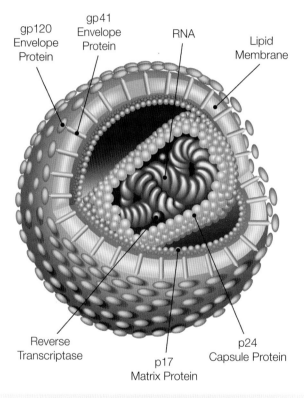

A virus. Chaga has strong antiviral properties, which are concentrated in alcohol extracts of wild chaga.

Chaga's Health Benefits

Research on chaga mushroom indicates that it provides the following benefits to human health:

Analgesic (removes pain)

Anodyne (soothes pain)

Antiallergenic

Antibacterial

Anticancer

Antihyperglycemic

Anti-inflammatory

Anti–lipid peroxidative (protects fats from oxidation or loss of electrons)

Antimutagenic

Antinociceptive (reduces sensitivity to painful stimuli)

Antioxidant

Antiparasitic (removes certain types of parasitic worms)

Antiplatelet aggregative effects (disperses clumped red blood cells)

Antitumor

Antiviral (flu, herpes, HIV, hepatitis)

Blood purifier

Blood sugar balancer

Cardioprotective

Fights bronchitis

Improves circulation

Immunomodulating

Induces apoptosis (the spontaneous breakdown of cancer cells)

Intestinal protection (good against colitis, gastritis, digestive inflammation)

Liver purification and detoxification

Lowers harmful LDL

Inotodiol and trametenolic acid, two of the primary bioactive compounds in chaga, show various biological activities, including antitumor, antiviral, antioxidant, and cytoprotective properties.[23] These compounds, along with chaga's extraordinary broad-spectrum nutrition profile, also help combat the mineral-deficiency/ toxicity/rancid oil/omega-6 overload syndrome we know as type 2 diabetes.

Chaga contains saponins (glycosides) of the triterpenoidal type. These unique triterpenes consist of three terpene units (terpenes are resins) attached to various types of sugar molecules, forming soaplike molecules where one side (the sugar) may attach to water, while the other side of the molecule (the triterpene) may attach to oil. Research indicates that these types of saponins have adaptogenic qualities: they improve immunity, lower LDL cholesterol, have anti-inflammatory effects, possess antioxidant activity, etc. Some saponins, such as astragaloside IV (found in the superherb astragalus) and gypenoside 49 (found in the superherb gynostemma), have radical genoprotective effects.

Chaga contains ergosterol, a precursor (or provitamin) to vitamin D_2 (ergocalciferol). Ultraviolet light turns ergosterol into viosterol, which is then converted into vitamin D_2. This is why when yeasts and mushrooms are exposed to ultraviolet light, vitamin D_2 is produced.[24] When dried in the sun, chaga contains vitamin D_2. Normally, vitamin D_3 (which is slightly different from D_2) is created in the skin under the influence of direct ultra-violet light and is then absorbed over the course of 24 to 36 hours.[25] However, in high-latitude winters, many people cannot get enough ultraviolet light on their bodies. Vitamin D is necessary for building new skin cells, as well as for bones, teeth, and hair. This vitamin regulates cell turnover and helps to control psoriasis. Vitamin D has been shown to help maximize the positive effects of antioxidant therapy and cancer drugs,[26] as well as to help protect against the development of multiple-sclerosis symptoms.[27] Even though vitamin D_3 is 3 to 9.5 times more potent than D_2 and has a longer duration of action, vitamin D_2 (found in chaga) is still an extraordinarily important nutrient.[28]

Korean Experts on Chaga

According to the Korean Nutrition Society, chaga:[29]

- increases the defense reactions of an organism
- stimulates metabolism in brain tissues
- has an anti-inflammatory effect when used internally and externally
- is an antioxidant
- delays the growth of some kinds of tumors
- lowers arterial and venous blood pressure
- regulates the heartbeat
- decreases sugar level in blood

Russian Experts on Chaga

According to the Russian Medical Academy, chaga:[30]

- has a positive effect against lung and liver cancer
- calms the nervous system

- is proven to positively affect various stomach diseases and ulcers
- stimulates the immune system

‹◦›

The Anticancer Arsenal

As we've seen, chaga has long been revered in Russia for its activity against cancer, both healing and protective. In the twelfth century Tsar Vladimir Monomah was treated with chaga (most probably for symptoms of lip cancer).[31] Chaga was approved for public use against cancer by the Medical Academy of Science in Moscow in 1955.

This folk-medicine wisdom continues to be proven valid by modern science. Many of chaga's anticancer properties are now being attributed to beta glucans, though of course this component works synergistically with the range of nutrients that chaga offers. Beta glucan is a type of medicinal, healing polysaccharide—a long-chain, nonsweet carbohydrate. It is a water-soluble nutrient and extracts in hot water (validating the use of chaga tea).

Because beta glucans usually occur in various types of clusters, the term is rarely used in the singular. Beta glucans are found in brewer's yeast, barley, oats, and seaweeds, and in more recent years have been discovered in the cell walls of bacteria and fungi, including reishi and chaga. Scientists and researchers have so far found twenty-nine types of beta glucans in chaga. *(Beta glucans are explored more fully in Part III.)*

Arguably, the most well-known Western research conducted on the use of chaga for health has been performed by Dr. Kirsti Kahlos and her team at the School of Pharmacology, University of Helsinki, Finland. Beginning in 1984, Dr. Kahlos's team conducted studies validating the immunomodulating impact of lanosterol-linked triterpenes as a flu vaccination and for antitumor applications. This research demonstrated that chaga has antiviral, antifungal, anticancer, and antitumor properties.[32]

Studies in Japan have determined the effectiveness of inotodiols (lanosterol compounds) in the destruction of mouse leukemia P388 cells.[33] Chaga inotodiols have also shown activity against carcinogens in mice.[34] And inotodiols have been shown to inhibit tumor growth in Balbc/c mice bearing Sarcoma-180 cells in vivo and to inhibit the growth in vitro of human carcinoma cell lines (lung carcinoma A-549 cells, stomach adenocarcinoma AGS cells, breast adenocarcinoma MCF-7 cells, and cervical adenocarcinoma HeLa cells).[35]

Furthermore, chaga is known to assist chemotherapy and other cancer treatments, probably for three primary reasons:

- Chaga's betulin is known to possess powerful liver-protective effects that help detoxify the chemotherapy chemicals and radiation damage.
- Chaga's extraordinary antioxidant properties very quickly squelch the strong oxidative damage to healthy tissue caused by radioactive chemotherapy.
- Chaga's melanin may bind radioactive isotopes into less toxic forms, allowing the detoxification of radioactive elements to occur.

Chemotherapy and Radiation Protection

Chaga is known to aid in the efficacy of chemotherapy and radiation treatments, and Solzhenitsyn's story of how he beat cancer with chaga and radiation treatments illustrates a famous example (related in *The Cancer Ward*). This may be due to chaga's melanin content: the pigment is also found in human skin as the component that makes skin darken from exposure to sunlight. Melanin has the propensity to bind radioactive isotopes into less toxic or even nontoxic forms. *(See pages 137–41 for more about melanin.)* Chaga has a particular affinity for fighting melanomas (skin cancer).

Chaga's support in chemotherapy can also be attributed to the King of Mushrooms' power to stop cancer cells from spreading by reinforcing and nourishing healthy cells, as well as preventing blood clumping and thrombi formation. Furthermore, chaga's joint usage with cancer-fighting pharmaceutical drugs and chemotherapy is known to diminish their side effects.[36]

Beta glucans have been shown to help assist chemotherapy and radiation treatments and to mitigate the damage caused by them.[37] Beta glucans are known to dramatically increase the body's ability to regenerate red blood cells following bone marrow injuries that occur from chemotherapy and radiation treatments.[38]

According to a study published in *Mutation Research* in 2003,

> This protective effect of beta-glucan could be attributed to its scavenging ability to trap free radicals produced during the biotransformation of these antineoplastic drugs [chemotherapy drugs that target rapidly dividing cells]. Beta-glucan also markedly restored the mitotic (cell division) activity of bone marrow cells that had been suppressed by the antineoplastic drugs. These results indicate that in addition to the known immunopotentiating activity of beta-glucan, it plays a role in reducing genotoxicity (capability to cause cancer) induced by antineoplastic drugs during cancer chemotherapy.[39]

In addition, beta glucans provides therapeutic support to prevent liver and kidney damage caused by the chemotherapy drug methotrexate.[40]

Chaga vs. Cancer

With its rich stores of triterpenes, unique minerals (cesium, rubidium, zinc, and germanium), and other beneficial nutrients, chaga appears to be effective in some way, shape, or form against all cancer and is particularly recommended for the following cancers:

Bone	Medulloblastoma
Brain	Melanoma
Breast	Neuroblastoma
Carcinoma	Ovarian
Cervical	Sarcoma (Ewing's)
Colon	Squamous cell cancers
Hepatoma	of the head and neck
Leukemia	Stomach
Liver	Uterine
Lung	

Cancer-Fighting Diets

It should be understood that not all advanced forms of cancer can be controlled, but chaga may still reduce pain, give comfort, and stop or slow cancerous growth. Some less advanced cases of cancer are arrested when caught early, and its spread (metastasis) may be prevented.

Prostate Cancer and Chaga

There is no direct evidence that chaga fights prostate cancer, only indirect evidence, since chaga's betulinic acid has been shown to fight prostate cancer.[41] In addition, chaga is known to suppress a stress-related chemical called nuclear factor B ("kappa B") that is associated with many cancers, including prostate cancer.[42]

Traditional Anticancer Chaga Diet

Anticancer chaga diets are traditionally restricted to milk products and vegetables—no meat/sausages, preservatives, or strong spices.[43] Chaga purifies the blood and regenerates deteriorated organs and glands.[44] Time must be allowed for chaga to work. The recommended treatment period is three to five months and is as follows: six to nine tablespoons (or two to three shots) of chaga alcohol tincture and eight cups of chaga tea per day. To make the tea, the bark and middle portion of wild chaga are thoroughly dried. It must then be crushed or shredded, and soaked in warm to hot water (not boiling). Per the traditional wisdom of using of chaga for cancer, think of it as yeast: water too hot will kill the living fungus.

In swelling of the lower bowel and in colon cancer, chaga decoctions are prepared for colonics.

Present-Day Anticancer Chaga Diet

The regimen below combines the best of the traditional approach to using chaga to control cancer with the best modern knowledge about nutrition. It is assumed that every item listed below is organic (grown without chemicals or sprays). Chemically treated food should be completely avoided when fighting cancer.

Chaga: Eight strong cups of wild chaga tea daily and/ or twenty to forty droppers full of chaga alcohol tincture each day. The chaga tincture should preferably be a dual extraction containing both the water-soluble and the alcohol-soluble fraction of wild chaga. While taking this or even greater dosages of tea or tincture, I recommend consuming other chaga products (e.g., capsules, dual extractions, mycelium, etc.), as well as other medicinal mushrooms, such as reishi, *Trametes versicolor,* maitake, shiitake,

Agaricus blazei, and *phellinus,* which have shown particular anticancer action.

Meat, poultry, fish: No meat or poultry (cooked or raw). Cooked salmon or trout (once or twice a week) may be consumed to maintain primordial strength (*jing* energy) and avoid wasting. Avoid commercially available sashimi (raw fish) due to tapeworm contamination.

Bread and crackers: No common bread. Instead, use raw chia, hempseed, and/or vegetable pulp crackers, as well as small amounts of Essene or Ezekial bread.

Dairy: Only fresh, raw butter and cultured goat's milk.

Fatty fruits: Avocados, olives. No sweet fruits, except some organic and wild berries in summer (no strawberries).

Oils: Fresh hempseed oil, olive oil (only the highest quality should be consumed), nonexcipient, non-solvent-extracted DHA/DPA/EPA algae oil, pharmaceutical-grade fish oil made from mackerel.

Fermented foods: Fresh, cultured kefir from raw goat's milk, nut mylk, or coconut water.

Raw egg yolks: The yellow egg yolk should be eaten raw or lightly cooked. It contains lecithin and sometimes DHA. The white of the egg contains strong enzyme inhibitors or antidigestive factors and should be discarded or eaten only if cooked.

Vegetables (cooked or raw): Green leafy vegetables should be especially favored, wild foods (sheep sorrel, red clover, malva/mallow leaf), and low-sugar, low-starch root vegetables. Celery-based, fresh, green vegetable juices are recommended.

Nuts: Eaten in moderation. Preferably either soak and dehydrate nuts or blend with pure spring water and then strain—the resulting liquid is known as a nut mylk. *(For more information on nut and seed mylks, see page 90).*

Seeds: Chia, hempseed, pumpkin, milk thistle. Soak and/or dehydrate seeds or blend your seeds with pure spring water and then strain to create a seed mylk. *(For more information on nut and seed mylks, see the Recipes section.)*

Seaweeds: All kinds.

Sprouts: No legume sprouts, only green sprouts such as broccoli, clover, alfalfa, etc.

Flowers: Red clover, passion flower, chamomile, rose, nasturtium, mallow flower, St. John's Wort, mint.

Superherbs: Chaga, reishi, maitake, shiitake, *Trametes versicolor, Agaricus blazei,* pau d'arco, cat's claw, sacha jergon, horsetail, nettle, neem, mangosteen rind, astragalus root, asparagus root, ginseng, schizandra berry, etc.

Superfoods: Marine phytoplankton, chlorella, bee pollen, royal jelly, noni powder, aloe vera gel, camu berry powder, unsweetened cacao in moderation, maca in moderation.

Supplements: Protocel, lysine, betaine (TMG), indole

3 carbinol with DIM, MegaHydrate, vitamin D_3, vitamin B_{12} (methylcobalamin), digestive and metabolic enzymes, Hawaiian or New Zealand sea salt.

Enemas: Chaga tea enemas once or twice daily. Wheatgrass juice enemas once or twice a week.

Fasting: Fasting on chaga tea is helpful and healing, as long as one's strength is good and wasting is not a problem. Fasting on chaga tea means eating no food and just drinking chaga tea.

Meanwhile, Back in the Cancer Ward

I'd like to close this part with another passage from Solzhenitsyn's novel *The Cancer Ward:*

> They all longed to find some miracle doctor, or some medicine the doctors here didn't know about. Whether they admitted as much or denied it, they all without exception in the depths of their hearts believed there was a doctor, or herbalist, or some old witch of a woman somewhere, whom you only had to find and get that medicine from to be saved.
>
> No, it wasn't possible, it just wasn't possible that their lives were already doomed.
>
> However much we laugh at miracles when we are strong, healthy and prosperous, if life becomes

so hedged and cramped that only a miracle can save us, then we clutch at this unique, exceptional miracle and believe in it!

And so Kostoglotov identified himself with the eagerness with which his friends were hanging on his lips and began to talk fervently, believing his own words even more than he'd believed the letter when he'd first read it to himself.

"Well, to start from the beginning. Sharaf, here it is. One of our old patients told me about Dr. Maslennikov. He said that he was an old pre-Revolutionary country doctor from the Alexandrov district near Moscow. He'd worked dozens of years in the same hospital, just like they used to do in those days, and he noticed that, although more and more was being written about cancer in medical literature, there was no cancer among the peasants who came to him. Now why was that?"

(Yes, why was that? Which of us from childhood has not shuddered at the mysterious? At contact with that impenetrable yet yielding wall behind which there seems to be nothing, yet from time to time we catch a glimpse of something which might be someone's shoulder, or else someone's hip? In our everyday, open, reasonable life, where there is no place for mystery, it suddenly flashes at us, 'Don't forget me! I'm here!')

"So he began to investigate, he began to investigate," repeated Kostoglotov. He never repeated anything, but now found pleasure in doing so. "And he discovered a strange thing: that the peasants in his district saved money on their tea, and instead of tea brewed up a thing call *chaga,* or in other words, birch fungus...."

"You mean brown cap?" Pudduyev interrupted him. In spite of the despair he'd resigned himself to and shut himself up in for the last few days, the idea of such a simple, easily accessible remedy burst upon him like a ray of light.

The people around him were all southerners, and had never in their lives seen a birch tree, let alone the brown-cap mushroom that grows under it, so they couldn't possibly know what Kostoglotov was talking about.

"No, Yefrem, not a brown cap. Anyway, it's not really a birch fungus, it's a birch cancer. You remember, on old birch trees there are these . . . peculiar growths, like spines, black on top and dark brown inside."

"Tree fungus, then?" Yefrem persisted. "They used to use it for kindling fires."

"Well, perhaps. Anyway, Sergei Nikitich Maslennikov had an idea. Mightn't it be that same *chaga* that had cured the Russian peasants of cancer for centuries without their even knowing it?"

"You mean they used it as a prophylactic?" The young geologist nodded his head.

Part II
Preparing and Enjoying Chaga

The first rule of superherbalism is compliance: will you actually take the superherbs? Will you ingest the chaga once you have it? That's why we now move into the fun of chaga picking and developing recipes to best consume it. If chaga hunting becomes enjoyable for you, then you will use chaga daily. If the chaga recipes you make taste great, you will drink it and/or eat it—and that is a key point.

Harvesting Your Own Wild Chaga

Marketing hype abounds concerning the supposed superiority of Siberian chaga versus chaga found in Finland or the United States or anywhere else. No research of which I am aware has systematically compared chaga samples from around the world for medicinal compounds, nutrients, and vitamins. However, chaga mineral content from worldwide samples have been compared *(see Chaga vs. Cancer: Let the Science Talk, on page 142)*. That research indicates that superior

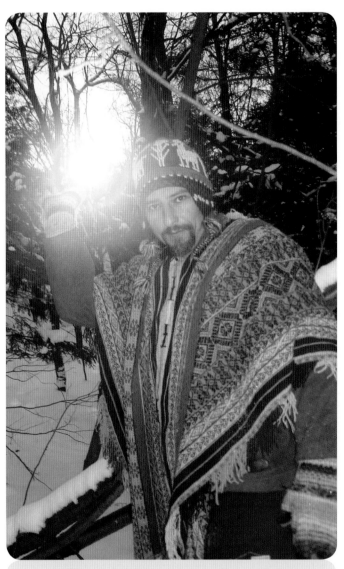

Late-season chaga hunting

chaga specimens are to be found within the forests of the Canadian Shield of eastern Canada.

Experience has shown me that old-growth forests containing birch tend to produce better-quality chaga specimens than do pioneering birch growth in post-deforested regions. This makes sense given the intact nature of a well-established mycelium community in a climax forest.

The best time to pick chaga mushroom is from mid-July to mid-November in the northern hemisphere. In cold winter temperatures, chaga sclerotia may become frozen to their tree and difficult to remove. Chaga hunting in winter requires a hatchet, whereas in summer, chaga hunting can be done by hand or with a large rock.

I prefer using my hands or a rock to remove the chaga conk (sclerotia) from its mother tree, because it feels more natural and keeps the tree healthier. (Metal hatchets are a shock to any tree due to the disturbing paramagnetic effect of the iron-steel on the wood.) The natural approach allows the tree to grow its chaga back more rapidly. Yes, over many years a chaga conk will typically grow back in the place on the tree where the chaga has been previously picked (if the tree lives on).

Often you will find chaga conks growing within reach as they emerge directly out of the side of a birch tree or near a large joint. However, many (including myself) have risked life and limb to collect chaga conks growing at heights greater than three meters up the tree. Leo Libman (a Russian mushroom researcher) says that traditionally (in Russia) they do not use wild chaga as a medicine unless it grows higher than 1.5 meters from the ground. Further inquiry into Libman's data (through my Finnish friend and fellow mushroom hunter Jaako Halmetoja) has indicated that the higher the chaga specimen is on the tree, the higher its concentration of medicinal betulin. (This data comes from Jaako and out-of-print Russian books by Leo Libman.)

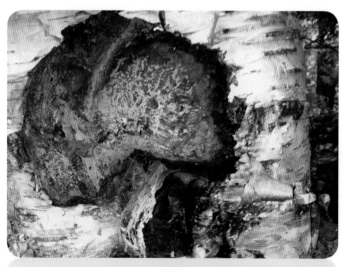

Chaga has just been picked from this birch by breaking it off by hand. No axe or saw was used.

Interestingly, the concentration and potency of different wild chaga mushrooms vary, depending on growing location, timing of the harvest, and the subsequent extraction method utilized to process them. In a 2008 study measuring the beta glucans content in chaga by different extraction and analytical methods, scientists found between 8.1g and 10.7g of beta glucans per 100g of the wild mushroom.[1]

Chaga Look-alikes: Often weak fungal infections that form cankers and burls on trees are mistaken for chagas. Also, be aware of a look-alike black fungi that grows predominantly on cherry, apricot, and plum

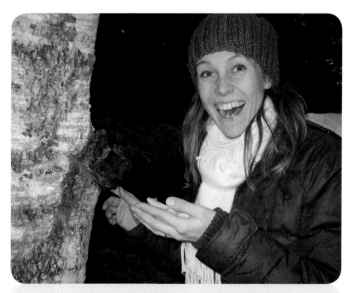

It is always a joy to find wild chaga.

trees in deciduous forests. It's known as *Apiosporina (Dibotryon) morbosa,* the black knot fungus. If you discover black knot fungi growing on any of your trees, be sure to cut or saw off the affected branch or twig and burn it to avoid infecting other trees.

Please be kind to the forest. Develop a relationship with the chaga life form. Be frugal with your chaga picking. The chaga conk is a prana-concentrating force in Nature. If all are picked, it is unknown what the complete effect will be. However, in my experience, I have felt that the subtle energy of the forest is disturbed from overharvesting chaga.

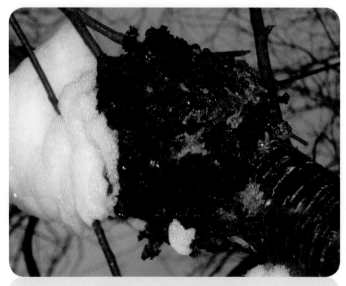

**The undesirable
black knot fungus**

Also, remember that chaga needs to be well dried after harvesting to avoid mold growth.

How to Store Wild Chaga

1. Dry the fresh, wild chaga in direct sunlight for several days. Bring the chaga in during the night and back out again during the day.
2. If the weather does not cooperate, dry the chaga in a dehydrator at a temperature of at least 105°F. Using a stove set at 200°F to 250°F also works and

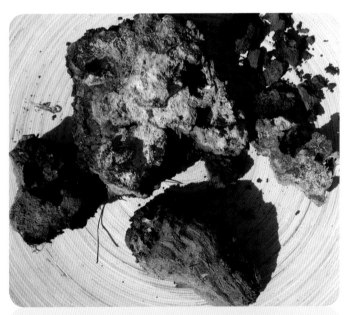

Sun-dried chaga chunks

dries the chaga faster than a dehydrator, although it's necessary to keep a close eye on the stove for several hours to avoid burning.

3. Break the chaga into golf ball–sized chunks with a mortar and pestle, or wrap the chaga in a small towel and gently break into chunks with a hammer against a hard surface.

   Store the completely dry chaga chunks in an airtight glass container (preferably Miron violet glass). If you live in a low-moisture home environment, put them in an open basket out on your kitchen table or, as is recommended in Russian folklore, store your dried chaga pieces and/or chaga products in a birch-bark box in order to enhance the subtle energies of chaga, which responds to its mother tree.

4. Use the chaga as needed. Since chaga is a tonic super-herb, I recommend taking some chaga every day that you eat or drink—especially if you live in a northern temperate climate. If a white film (mildew) begins to develop on the outer black bark of the chaga, that piece may still be good for tea, but it must be used immediately. Avoid storing chaga if it already has this white mildew film. This type of white mildew is not present on wild chaga. It is something that can attack chaga that has already been picked and dried incorrectly (trapping moisture that mildew can use as a growth medium).

Chaga Products on the Market

Several types of chaga products exist in the world market:

- Wild chaga: This is wild, naturally growing chaga sclerotium picked from a tree (usually birch). Wild chaga specimens are typically dried and distributed; yet they may also be crushed into a powder and distributed in that form.

- Techno-grown chaga powders (usually sold in capsules in health-food stores and online): These products come from laboratory-controlled chaga mycelium grown on grain material (usually organic

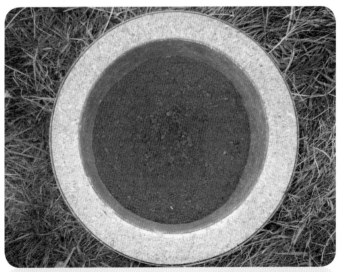

Dried, wild chaga powder may be eaten as food or with food.

rice). Raw mycelium products are preferable. The idea of making mycelium more bio-available by heat, alcohol, and chemical processing does not necessarily improve mycelium products. Mushroom proteins and enzymes begin to be broken down by heat above 150°F (65°C). The proteins and enzymes are also broken down by alcohol and strong bases such as sodium hydroxide. In the raw mycelium, most of the beneficial enzymes are intact. These include glucoamylase, laccase, peroxidase, protease, superoxide dismutase, etc. Furthermore, mycelium cell walls are made of chitin fibrils in a protein and polysaccharide matrix. The chitin content averages about 12% of the cell wall material. This is too small a composition of chitin to require heat extraction of the polysaccharide fraction of the mycelium. The raw chaga mycelium should preferably be freeze-dried. If you can, avoid oxidized spray-dried products, although they are better than nothing. The techno-grown mycelium of chaga contains more protein and several different polysaccharides compared to wild chaga. Again, these techno-grown mushrooms comprise many of the encapsulated chaga and mushroom products, with some exceptions.

- Hot-water extracts of chaga: This includes chaga tea and certain encapsulated chaga products. Hot water extracts most of chaga's polysaccharides, including immune-balancing beta glucans.

- Chaga alcohol extracts: Chaga's medicinal liver-protective, tumor-fighting, cancer-fighting triterpenes and betulin-family molecules are alcohol-soluble.

- Chaga extracts consisting of mixtures of both alcohol and hot-water extracts: These are often called "dual extracts" because they use two mediums of extraction.

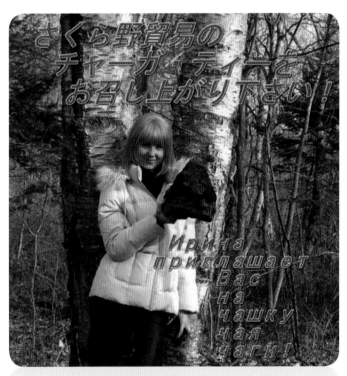

A Russian advertisement for chaga

- Extracted, fermented chaga mycelium or sclerotia: This involves using bacteria to break down the chaga into different and perhaps more active, smaller biological units. Of the fermented chaga products, chaga *jun* cultures are the most familiar to me. *Jun* is a bacterial culture, similar in concept to kombucha, yet without yeast and fungal components. This type of product is usually not commercially available, but it can be made at home by alchemists, scientists, and food researchers.

- Chaga medicines: These are products that I have no familiarity with except by reading about them. One is called "Bifungen," a refined extract of chaga that has been used in Russia since 1955 for the treatment of stomach and intestinal diseases.[2]

Commonly Used Kitchen Equipment

Here are a few key items specified and commonly used in these recipes.

Stove Choices

My experience has taught me that wood-burning stoves produce the best heat for making tea. Not only does a wood-burning stove heat the cookware upon its metal surface, but it also produces infrared heat. The infrared heat released by the burning wood inside the stove heats the water uniquely and fairly uniformly. Infrared heat appears to me to provide a better overall extraction of polysaccharides, minerals, and other active ingredients out of mushrooms, roots, and barks.

A reasonable water-heating choice is gas flame heat. This is typical in present-day homes. This is the type of flame that is fueled by natural gas, propane, kerosene, or another type of flammable gas. The open flame creates some infrared heat, yet most of the heating comes from the contact of the plasma flame to the cookware, which in turn heats the water.

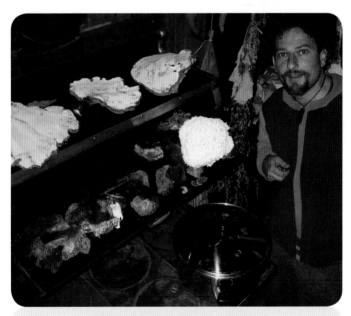

There's nothing like a wood-burning stove.

Magnetic inductance coil technology provides for an interesting way to heat water with diminished dangers of accidentally losing control of fire or burning oneself. This system uses a magnetic field to heat the metal of the kettle. Only the kettle becomes hot, and that in turn heats the water inside. This type of system is made available by Saladmaster Inc. and uses a kettle made of the highest quality, non-outgassing, 316T stainless steel. Like most kitchen appliances such as toasters and coffeemakers, magnetic coil heaters and ceramic electric cookpots do emit dirty electromagnetism (unnatural electromagnetic fields originating in the electricity in the home that gets amplified by the appliance and projected outward into the tea and perhaps into you—even if you are not touching the appliance).

The last choice is electric stove heat—these are commonly found in homes all over Western civilization. Electric burners heat the cookware, which in turn heats the water. Very little infrared heat is generated. Like magnetic coil heaters and ceramic cookpots, electrical-coil heaters produce heat that carries dirty electromagnetic energy from the electricity into your cookware and tea.

I personally use a non-outgassing, 16-liter Salad-Master 316T Stainless Steel cookware pot on my wood-burning stove. That is what I have determined to be ideal for large-scale tea making.

Blender

An average blender is capable of doing most of the recipes you find in this book. However, due to the low power, a normal blender is other than ideal. A high-powered blender is best when you want to liquify your drinks completely. A high-powered blender such as the Nutri-Bullet Nutrient Extractor is a great addition to any active chaga-processing kitchen. A high-powered blender can pulverize an entire dried chaga into a powder. I don't necessarily recommend that; I feel you keep more of chaga's nutrients intact by crushing it to a powder with mortar and pestle than with the spinning blades of metal. However, you have to use the tools you have in the time you have.

Mortar and Pestle

This is an item pair for all wild-chaga hunters, super-herb growers, and wild-food enthusiasts. I recommend getting a large granite mortar and pestle with an approximately 7-inch (18-cm) inner bowl diameter and a 9-inch (23-cm) outer diameter. That will be big enough to crush and grind dried chaga. You can usually obtain these in the Chinatown shopping areas of any major city.

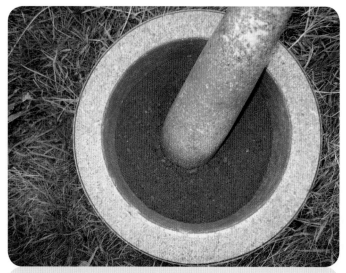

The indispensable mortar and pestle

The Double-Boiler System

Several of the chaga recipes and extraction techniques in this book call for using the double-boiler technique to melt hardened oils such as cacao butter. Using a double-boiler system to do this works great. Fill a pot halfway with water and then put a heat-resistant Mason glass jar or Pyrex (boro-silicate) container filled with your hardened oil inside the pot of water. Heat the pot up and wait for the hardened oil to melt, at which point you are ready to extract herbal substances within the hot melted oil or to simply pour and use the liquefied oil.

Types of Water and Mycelium

Where I mention water, I recommend that you use fresh spring water. As a distant second, you can use the best purified water you can find. Tap water is too polluted and should be avoided.

Coconut water may also be used (not for tea making, but for blending into beverages), and fortunately, coconut water is becoming a more common option. If you live in the temperate woodlands where chaga grows, you may also use maple water (maple water is boiled down to make maple syrup) or birch water (birch water is boiled down to make birch syrup).

Many of the medicinal mushroom products on the market consist primarily of rice-grown mycelium that have been dried, powdered, and encapsulated; although some are hot-water extracts turned into powder or other types of alchemical extraction mixtures.

In the old days, we had to open individual capsules when making recipes. Today bulk mycelium powders, including chaga mycelium, are becoming increasingly available, making everyone's life easier (see www .longevitywarehouse.com). If all you have is capsules, typically five or six 500-milligram capsules will provide one tablespoon of mycelium powder.

◄○►

Mixing Chaga with Other Herbs and Medicinal Mushrooms

Unless one has allergies to mushrooms, one may consume a variety of medicinal mushrooms simultaneously to get a wide variety of polysaccharides and beta glucans for an enhanced immunological effect. This "guilding" of different medicinal mushrooms together creates what mushroom expert Paul Stamets terms a "host defense"—an immunological defense barrier against illness.

Guilding superherbs and chaga together has similar effects: the immune system is fortified by saponins, polysaccharides, and other nutrients from various superherbs that assist the chemistry of chaga.

One might wonder if there is a problem with combining all these herbs—such as the theory of proper food combining might tell us. The answer is a tentative "no." I tend to stick to traditional herbal formulas or vary them slightly. Herbal miscombining can happen, yet typically it will not cause indigestion; instead, poor results, unfavorable flavors, and/or minor toxic effects will emerge.

It's smart to respect and defer to ancient herbal combination strategies. These systems were arrived at through thousands of years of practice and intuition. Traditional herbal formulas are a solid and trustworthy foundation, though breaking the rules and experimenting with updated herb combinations is recommended, because even in failure it is fun, and new innovations are required in our world today.

Generally, in herbalism, a primary herb is selected. This is supported by a second and third herb that help to deliver, enhance, and balance the primary herb.

A typical and traditional chaga tea combination might contain: chaga (primary herb), birch polypore (secondary herb), and nettle (tertiary herb). An updated chaga tea combination might contain: chaga (primary herb), astragalus (secondary herb), and goji berry (tertiary herb). Of course, you can go beyond three herbs in a combination or arrange the herbs in any fashion you wish.

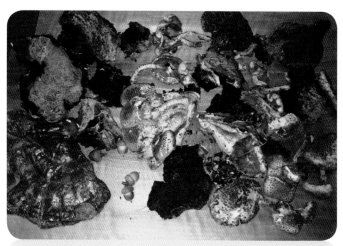

Reishi, chaga, and *Pholiota* mushrooms

Recipes

One of the main goals of this book is to give you tools to improve health as well as fight infections and cancer while still enjoying your foods and beverages. Chaga opens up many options. The information and recipes in this section are designed to help us more easily create and utilize every type of chaga product.

As always, I recommend eating organic foods and raw foods (due to their superior concentration of nutrients), so the assumption in every recipe is that the ingredients are raw and organic, unless they cannot be made raw (e.g., maple syrup) or are specified otherwise.

A Note about Sweeteners

In these recipes I primarily recommend using "normal" or relatively common sweeteners such as honey and maple syrup. Or you can use low-glycemic sweeteners including lucuma, *lo han guo* (sweetener made from a fruit and used in Chinese medicine) and/or exotic birch syrup (if you can find it!). Dried fruits such as figs, goji berries, and dates soaked in pure water also make great moderate-glycemic sweeteners that you can experiment with. Try variations using the rehydrated fruits and/or their soak water (the soak water will be low-glycemic).

One thing we know about sugar—sugar feeds infections and cancer. Therefore, if you have infections such as candida, hepatitis, and cancer, it makes sense to avoid all sweeteners with the exceptions of completely nonglycemic xylitol and stevia.

Xylitol

"Xylitol looks, tastes, and feels exactly like sugar; however, chemically speaking, xylitol is not actually a sugar, but a sugar alcohol. Unlike other sweeteners such as sorbitol, fructose, and glucose, the xylitol molecule has five instead of six carbon atoms. As a five-carbon sugar, xylitol has antimicrobial properties, whereas six-carbon sugars can cause bacterial and fungal overgrowths.

"Xylitol is actually so natural that our bodies constantly produce 5 to 15 grams per day under normal metabolism conditions. The natural presence of xylitol in plants, food, and humans suggests that consuming xylitol (in reasonable quantities) is safe for our health. Commercially obtainable xylitol is not a raw, whole-food product; however, xylitol itself is a natural substance.

"When choosing xylitol products, I recommend seeking out only birch-derived xylitol."

—FROM THE LONGEVITYNOW PROGRAM[3]

Teas

If you really want to dive into chaga's medicinal and spiritual powers, drink three to eight cups of chaga tea daily, preferably on an empty stomach and before meals.

Chaga contains no stimulants (no caffeine or other methylxanthines such as theophylline or theobromine). It can be a great morning or late-evening tea. It may be consumed hot or cold in any season. Chaga tea's general humor (from the Galen perspective) is that it is hot (increases body heat) and dry (balances those who are too internally damp); however, as a superherb, it has adaptogenic qualities and refits itself to support the specific character of the person.

Preparing Chaga Tea

One would use wild chaga—not lab-grown chaga mycelium—to make tea. Generally the more surface area of wild chaga sclerotia you expose (the more you crush the wild chaga into a powder), the greater the extraction you will get into the medium you are working with (e.g., water, alcohol, oil, etc.).

Contrary to some opinions, chaga does not have to be boiled to make a delicious, alkaline, medicinal tea.

The extraordinarily rich melanin pigments found in chaga, as well as its polysaccharides, are extracted into water when chaga tea is made. In addition, chaga contains vanillic acid, which comes through into the tea. These elements produce a wild-mushroom tea that looks like maple syrup and has hints of vanilla. It is unlike any other tea in the world!

Here are the steps:

1. After finding an appropriate teapot (I recommend 316T stainless steel cookware or Pyrex glass) and a strainer, you are ready to begin your tea-making.

2. Fill your teapot with pure cold water. Start by putting your ground chaga (or chaga chunks), herbs and/or tea bag(s) in this water. Allow the herbs to soak in the water (steep). Before heating at all, you can steep the herbs cold for a few minutes up to an hour.

3. Although it can be done more swiftly, take the cold water up to a hot temperature (no hotter than three-quarters of the way to a full boil) in 45 minutes to 1 hour. This allows for a better extraction of herbal ingredients and essences. You never have to fully boil the tea.

4. Use the strainer and push it into the tea surface to push all the chaga chunks away. Dip a ladle into the area within the strainer and enjoy!

What about renewing the tea? When should the tea be thrown away and restarted? Chaga, like all wild mushrooms, dense roots, and barks, can stay in the tea for days—even over a week as long as you keep a lid on the tea when the tea is cool.

What type of water should you use? Of course, all municipal tap water anywhere in the world should be assiduously avoided (except for Reykjavik, Iceland). Preferentially, for all herbal tea-making, use spring water with a low TDS (total dissolved solids) and low calcium and iron content. Preferably collect your own spring water from local sources (try www.findaspring .com) or acquire the best spring water bottled in glass you can get your hands on. Purified and distilled water are lesser options, yet may serve the purpose when other options are not available.

Avoid boiling. Three-quarters to boiling (160°F or 75°C) is as hot as your tea water needs to be in order to extract all the active water-soluble compounds in barks and roots.

Even though very hot, boiling water has slightly more capability than cooler temperatures of water to extract alcohol and fat-soluble compounds (therefore extracting more compounds from the chaga), I disagree with the entire concept of boiling, because it damages water. Paul Kouchakoff's research[4] on white blood cell reactions indicates that boiling water or bringing it to a near boil disturbs the water molecules so dramatically that even after the water is cooled down and consumed, it will cause a white blood cell reaction in the drinker as if s/he ate cooked food. This white blood cell response does not appear when one ingests raw food or water that has not exceeded three-quarters of the way to boiling (160°F or 75°C). This white blood cell response theoretically indicates that boiled water and/or cooked foods cause biological confusion and thus activate the immune system.

Russian Chaga Tea

The following Russian chaga tea is perhaps the most written-about method on the Internet of making tea from wild chaga. Why do it this way? I don't know. I include it for novelty purposes.

1. Break up the dried chaga mushroom into chunks.
2. Soak a few of these chaga chunks in cold water for four hours.
3. Filter with a strainer and save the liquid and the soft, wet chaga chunks separately.
4. Pour water heated to a temperature of about 50°C (122°F) over the softened chaga in a ratio of five parts water to one part chaga.
5. Let stand at room temperature for 48 hours.
6. Filter the new mixture and add this water to that prepared in step 3.
7. Use this batch within four days, drinking three glasses at eight-hour intervals each day. After four days make a new batch of chaga tea.

Chaga Superbowl Boil Tea

The following tea recipe comes from some folks on the Internet who say that boiling the chaga releases additional cancer-fighting ingredients which we now understand to be slightly more fat-soluble triterpenes. Even though this conflicts with my own perceptions about the problems with boiling, I include it because it is something you may want to try in order to determine the effects for yourself:

1. Put two to three handfuls of chaga mushroom chunks into a container of 2 gallons (8 liters) or more.
2. Pour in just under 2 gallons (8 liters) of water.
3. Cover the pot.
4. Heat the water to a roiling boil for several hours.
5. Drink the chaga tea hot, warm, or after it cools.
6. Even after boiling, the chaga chunks can be used over and over.

Maximizing Wild Chaga Tea Extractions

To improve your chaga extraction, it is recommended that you freeze your chaga tea (containing the chaga pieces) after hot-water extraction. Once the chaga tea and pieces are frozen, they are to be reheated. The freezing is intended to break down as much fiber in the chaga pieces as possible, thus liberating the most medicinal elements when the chaga is reheated.

Many liver-supporting, cancer-fighting, and tumor-fighting triterpenes and betulin compounds are alcohol-soluble but not necessarily water-soluble. Therefore, in order to maximize your wild chaga extraction, a fraction of your wild chaga should be crushed and put in an alcohol-based medium containing at least 40% alcohol (a higher percentage of alcohol is better). One can also repurpose spent chunks of chaga used for tea making: simply dry the spent chunks out in a dehydrator or stove and then, when cool and dry, take the spent chunks and drop them into alcohol. I recommend using alcohol that is over 120 proof so that it is strong enough to act as an effective solvent of chaga's alcohol- and fat-soluble medicines.

Chaga alcohol tinctures may be added to teas, food, or beverages, or may be consumed directly.

◄◦►

Nut and Seed Mylks

You may want to enjoy your chaga tea with a creamer. If you use dairy products, I recommend purchasing organic, raw dairy. A simpler alternative to a dairy creamer is nut and seed mylks. To make these tasty creamers, simply soak your nuts or seeds in water overnight, then blend with pure spring water (or more chaga tea) and strain—the resulting liquid is known as a nut or seed mylk.

If you want to take your creation one step further, you can blend in pitted low-glycemic dried fruits (such as prunes), as well as some vanilla powder. If you want to go further, culture your nut or seed mylk in a pitcher by adding 2,000 to 3,000 mg of probiotic or kefir powder. Stir with a wooden spoon. Place a clean rag over the top of the pitcher and secure with a rubber band. Let the pitcher stand for 24 to 36 hours at room temperature. Agitate the pitcher every couple of hours to keep the probiotic culture mixing and active. After the nut or seed mylk has fermented, refrigerate. You now have a nut- or seed-mylk kefir.

◄◦►

Alcohol Extracts

Although we now see it everywhere, distilled, pure, high-proof (80+ proof) alcohol is actually an alchemical product that is difficult to produce without the required skills, experience, and materials. My research indicates that in our historical era, European alchemists during the Middle Ages were the first to develop high-proof alcohol. This substance can extract alcohol-soluble and fat-soluble compounds such as the cancer-fighting lanostanes and other triterpenes in chaga, whereas even very hot water (which has more fat-soluble extraction properties than water at cooler temperatures) still cannot significantly extract these compounds. Therefore, alcohol tinctures allow us to access medicines in herbs that we normally do not extract via hot water or even through digestion.

How to Make a Chaga Tincture

1. On the new moon, put two to four heaping table-spoons of powdered wild chaga into 0.5 liter alcohol. The alcohol can range from vodka strength (80 to 100 proof) all the way to pure organic ethanol, at 190 proof. I recommend alcohol that is 120+ proof for chaga extracts.
2. Place the chaga with the alcohol in a sealed container and shake daily until the full moon (or any subsequent full moon).

3. On the full moon, filter out the chaga particles using a fine mesh strainer. The remaining alcohol liquid is your chaga extract.

4. Mix down the chaga extract so as to bring the proof of the final tincture to 60 to 70 proof (30% to 35% alcohol). For example, if you are using 100-proof vodka to extract the chaga, you will have to add spring or purified water to dilute the tincture after the extraction phase. The amount of water you add is two-thirds the volume of the 100-proof extract. Basically, you are diluting the extract until it is 60 proof.

5. Pour off into dropper bottles.

A Drop of Chaga for Every Year of Life

"The Minnesota Mycological Society had a fungus exhibit at the Science Museum of Minnesota. There was a big chunk of chaga on the table. One of the visitors was a Russian physician. She immediately recognized it and enthusiastically told us about how it is used in her country. The chaga is used as a very concentrated alcohol tincture. The prescription: give three times daily one drop of tincture for each year of the patient's age. That would be 62 drops for me!"

— RON SPINOSA, "THE CHAGA STORY,"
THE MYCOPHILE 47, NO. 1

For a healthy person, the appropriate chaga alcohol tincture dosage is 3 to 6 full droppers per day. For those requiring herbal assistance to improve health, this dosage can be significantly increased to as high as 20 to 40 full droppers per day.

In a personal email to me dated January 5, 2010, one of the world's leading mushroom scientists, Paul Stamets, wrote the following concerning mushroom chemistry extraction methods:

> Water extraction can pull out most heavy molecular-weight polysaccharides (immunopotentiators). Ethanol extraction can pull out many sterols (antivirals), triterpenoids (anti-inflammatories), and ergothioneines (antioxidants). CO_2 extraction pulls out lipids and other fatty acids (immunopotentiators)... and the list of solvents (acetone, hexane, benzene, DMSO) that can be used for extracting polar and non-polar compounds is extensive, depending upon what your target is.
>
> Each extraction method separates one group of constituents away from the medicinal matrix. The isolated constituent may not confer the same health benefit as the whole—one of the tenets of integrative medicine.
>
> The original research on PSK, for instance, was from mycelium not fruitbodies. As the mycelium matures, building-block sugars are constructed.

We [Fungi Perfecti] grow our mycelium to early fruitbody, the primordial stage, so we benefit from both. The vast majority of cordyceps products, for instance, also come from mycelium, as are most of the Turkey Tail products (despite what others may say).

Oil Extracts

Because I do not yet have a CO_2 extraction device, I have resorted to cruder forms of extracting fat-soluble substances from chaga. I crush wild, dried chaga to a powder with a large granite mortar and pestle (again, I prefer this to coffee grinders and blenders). I then typically mix the resulting chaga powder with a combination of the following raw, organic oils (totaling 0.10 liter): coconut oil 30%, cacao butter 30%, olive oil 30%, hempseed oil 10%. I will add anywhere from 25 to 50 grams of powdered wild chaga and sometimes other substances that I like to get fat-soluble extracts from (e.g., fresh *Mucuna pruriens* beans). All the oil and the chaga and any other herbs go into a Pyrex (boro-silicate) container or a large jar (without the lid). I then place this container into a pot of water.

This setup is known as a double-boiler system (as described previously). The stove heats the water up in the first container (the saucepan or cooking pot), which in turn heats up the oil slowly and gently in the second container (the jar or Pyrex container), allowing the chaga to extract into the oil. You can let this system run for hours as long as you keep an eye on your stove and refill the water occasionally. This is a wonderful system when you have a wood-burning stove because of the extraction benefits of the infrared heat.

Chaga oil extracts can be used for salad dressings, hot teas (add the chaga-infused oil into the hot tea— this is delicious if you use only cacao butter as the oil), homemade chocolate creations, and homemade liniments of all types.

I have done no scientific testing on chaga oil extracts and have found nothing in the literature. Personally, I have felt strong adrenal-kidney-*jing*-building effects from consuming chaga-infused oils. Because chaga has such an affinity for the skin, it would make sense to put the oil extract into homemade skincare products. More research is required in this area.

Chaga Oil Exfoliating Body Scrub

(recipe by Andrea McGinnis)

Mix the following ingredients together in a Mason jar or similar container (such as Pyrex) that can fit into a double-boiler system.

- 1/4 cup chaga powder (you can also use whole chaga ground up very fine with a mortar and pestle)
- 1/2 cup raw cold-pressed virgin coconut oil
- 1/4 cup raw cacao butter or cacao paste
- 1/4 cup raw cold-pressed extra-virgin olive oil
- 1/4 cup nontoasted sesame oil
- 1 1/2 cups finely granulated sea salt or pink Himalayan salt (you can also use raw organic cane sugar or a combination of both)
- 1 teaspoon vitamin E oil
- 1 tablespoon jojoba oil
- 20 to 30 drops of essential oils of your choice (make sure they are organic/wildcrafted). Some combinations might include: sandalwood, rose, vetiver, vanilla, frankincense or lemongrass, and mint or orange, patchouli, ginger or ylang ylang, jasmine, rose, lavender or rosemary, bergamot, clary sage, cedar. Be creative!

Heat all these items together using a double-boiler system (place the container with all the ingredients within a deep pan filled with water). Heat the outer pan, which in turn heats the inner container of oils. Avoid placing a lid on the oil-filled container.

To utilize this chaga body scrub, get your skin wet first via a warm shower or sauna. Then use a natural exfoliating brush to scrub the mixtures all over your body. Wait 10 to 20 minutes before rinsing off (the longer you let the chaga soak in, the better).

Enjoy the beta glucan glow!

Chaga Beverages

From an herbal-shamanic perspective, chaga is in some strange way a temperate-climate energetic-value equivalent to tropical cacao (chocolate). Chaga lives in colder temperate forests instead of tropical jungles, where cacao originates. Both contain mineral-rich fibers, medicinal properties, and extraordinary antioxidant levels, along with a palette of other nutrients. Both chaga and cacao have been traditionally consumed as beverages. Chaga beverages are explored in this section . . . and keep in mind that the combination of cacao and chaga is truly a gustatory, culinary, and nutritional marvel.

Chaga Coffee

1 liter wild chaga tea

1/4 liter almond mylk

1 tablespoon honey, maple syrup, birch syrup,
   or xylitol (optional)

The almond mylk can be purchased in health-food stores. Follow the nut- and seed-mylk instructions *(see page 90)* to make your own almond mylk. Store the almond mylk in the refrigerator until use. Blend or stir all ingredients and serve. In Finland, during World War II, chaga was used as a replacement for coffee due to food rationing.

Serves: 2

Fermenting Chaga

When I first began experimenting with chaga mushroom conks, we created a chaga *jun* (a fermented beverage somewhat similar to kombucha). The beverage was interesting in flavor and effect. If one has strong strains (bacterial cultures) of probiotic microorganisms, wild chaga can be fermented. Chaga can be added to yogurts and kefirs made with raw cow's milk, raw goat's milk and/or raw nut mylk.

Summer Blueberry Chaga Surprise

4 ounces fresh or frozen blueberries

1 heaping tablespoon hempseed butter

1/3 blender full hempseed mylk

2 tablespoons reishi mycelium

1 to 2 tablespoons wild honey, maple syrup,
   birch syrup, or xylitol

2 to 3 teaspoons vanilla extract

1 tablespoon astragalus extract powder

1 liter cold chaga tea

The hempseed mylk can be purchased in health-food stores or made by blending hempseed with cold pure water *(see page 90)*. When the mylk is ready, put all the ingredients in a blender. Fill the rest of the blender up with the cold chaga tea. Blend and *voilà!* Drink and go wild in the forest. Blueberries improve eyesight and activate the brain. Hempseed is an overall body tonic containing omega-3 ALA fatty acids and omega-6 GLA anti-inflammatory fatty acids, along with a complement of complete globular edestin protein. Reishi and astragalus nourish the immune system and increase longevity. Chaga delivers its magic on top of all this.

Serves: 2 to 3

Chaga Huang-Qi

- 1 liter wild chaga and astragalus tea
- 1 tablespoon chaga mycelium
- 1 tablespoon astragalus extract
- 2 tablespoons lysine powder
- 1 tablespoon wild honey, maple syrup, birch syrup, or xylitol (optional)

Use wild chaga for the tea. The astragalus you use for the tea can be the bulk product you buy from Chinese herb shops and that looks like a tongue depressor. Make the tea.

In a separate blender, put the chaga mycelium, astragalus extract, and optional sweetener. Preferably select FITT brand astragalus extract, available at www.longevitywarehouse.com. Chaga and astragalus are two of the most powerful herbs in the world. Together they help you connect (to Nature) and protect (your tissues) while you select (the frequency of genius). The lysine is added as a potent cancer-, virus-, and infection-fighting amino acid that helps build bone density.

Serves: 2

Double Chaga, Double Reishi Espresso

   1 liter of wild chaga and wild reishi tea

   1 tablespoon chaga mycelium

   1 tablespoon reishi mycelium

   3 droppers full of chaga alcohol tincture (extract)

   1 tablespoon honey, maple syrup, birch syrup,
      or xylitol (optional)

Place the mycelium, chaga tincture, and sweetener(s) of choice in your blender. Pour in the hot, warm, or cold tea (depending on your preference). Blend and serve. Chaga is king and reishi is queen. Together they enrobe you in majesty.

Serves: 2

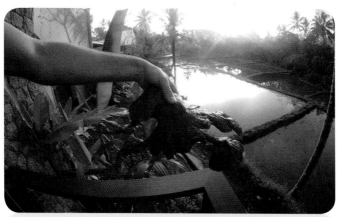

Photo by Sage Dammers

A reishi mushroom in Bali

Elegy to Bubbling Springs

2 liters of wild chaga, birch polypore,
   Fomes fomentarius, reishi, *Pholiota* spp.
   (or shiitake or maitake), birch bark, and
   tsugae-pine (hemlock-pine tree) needle
   tea made in fresh spring water

2 tablespoons chaga mycelium

2 tablespoons reishi mycelium

2 tablespoons phycocyanin (the blue pigments
   from spirulina or AFA blue-green)

2 tablespoons wild honey, maple syrup, birch
   syrup, or xylitol

The key to this recipe, of course, is finding all the wild mushrooms to make the tea. Ideally these should all be sourced in temperate climate areas near natural cold-water springs. Use just a fingerstrip of birch bark and five to eight pine needles. Place the dry ingredients (mycelium, phycocyanin) and honey in a blender. If the mushroom flavor aspects of the tea are strong, the honey will take the edge off. Pour the hot, warm, or cool mushroom tea into the blender (however you prefer it) and blend with the other ingredients. This recipe is designed to deliver levitative Ormus minerals while activating super immunity.

Serves: 3

Divine Chaga Chai

(Recipe by Andrea McGinnis)

6 to 8 liters chaga tea (steep for at least 2 hours)

Bring tea to a low simmer, turn off heat, and add the following herbs (feel free to add more/less to achieve an inspired taste!). Then steep again for 30 minutes.

1/2 of a star anise

10 to 12 whole dried clove flowers

6 to 7 whole allspice berries

1 heaping teaspoon of tea-cut cinnamon bark (or 2 short sticks)

6 to 7 whole white peppercorns

1 cardamom pod opened to the seeds

1 freshly grated nutmeg

2 whole vanilla beans, sliced open

In a blender, place the following ingredients:

1 to 3 tablespoons honey, maple syrup, birch syrup, or xylitol

1 to 3 tablespoons raw nut butter to taste (almond, pecan, macadamia, Brazil, cashew, etc.)

2 to 3 tablespoons lucuma powder (optional)

1 to 2 tablespoons maca powder (optional)

Pour the hot, warm, or cold strained tea mixture into the blender. Blend well and enjoy!

Serves: 5 to 6

Quick Chocolate Chaga Charge-Up!
(Recipe by Andrea McGinnis)

  2 liters spring water
  1 cup raw organic hempseeds (add more hemp
     for a thicker mylk)

Blend in a high-speed blender on high for approximately 20 seconds. Strain mylk through a nut-mylk bag. In the blender add to the mylk:

  2 tablespoons organic raw cacao powder
  2 to 3 tablespoons honey (to taste) or
     your sweetener of choice
  1 teaspoon vanilla powder or extract
  1 teaspoon raw organic virgin coconut oil
  1 teaspoon raw cacao butter
  1/4 teaspoon sea salt
  2 tablespoons chaga mycelium powder
  1 to 2 tablespoons maca powder
  1 to 2 teaspoons carob powder
  1 to 2 teaspoons mesquite powder
  1 to 2 teaspoons powdered *ho shou wu* (fo-ti)*
     (optional)
  1 to 3 teaspoons of medicinal mushroom powders,
     such as reishi, cordyceps, lion's mane, agaricus,
     shiitake, maitake, tremella, etc. (optional)

Blend ingredients together on high for 20 seconds. To serve chilled, add a few spring-water ice cubes and blend again until frothy.

Serves: 3 to 4

෴

Superfood Superherbal

(Recipe by Adam Collins of SuperfoodSnacks.com)

1 tablespoon chaga mycelium powder

3/4 cup fresh blueberries

1 to 2 tablespoons raw honey

11/2 liters coconut water, or hemp or almond mylk

1 tablespoon raw cacao butter

1 tablespoon bee pollen

4 to 6 capsules pearl powder**

1/2 teaspoon LongevityWarehouse.com's marine phytoplankton

1/2 teaspoon of *ho shou wu*

1/2 teaspoon ashwaganda powder

1/2 teaspoon camu camu powder

1/2 teaspoon maca powder

Ho shou wu (sometimes *he shou wu* or misnamed as *fo-ti*) is a Chinese yin *jing* longevity, bone-marrow, kidney-adrenal superherb.

**Pearl powder is commonly used in Chinese and Persian longevity medicine. It was also part of the ancient Egyptian system of medicine.

Here we have the most powerful superherbs mixed with the most powerful superfoods. This one should activate dormant superhero powers. Blend everything together to perfection and enjoy!

Serves: 4 to 6

Superhero Chaga Activator

(Recipe by Adam Collins of SuperfoodSnacks.com)

1 thumb-sized chunk of chaga

1 heaping tablespoon horsetail

1 heaping tablespoon nettles

1 heaping tablespoon *ho shou wu*

1 tablespoon oatstraw

1 tablespoon pau d'arco

1 tablespoon cat's claw

1/2 vanilla bean

Put all these dried herbs into a pot. Then fill the pot with 1 gallon (4 liters) of water. Avoid boiling. Just set the burner on a low setting and heat it up. Ideally you're looking for about 150°F (65°C).

Next, place in a blender the following ingredients:

1 tablespoon maca powder

5 tablespoons raw cacao powder

5 tablespoons lucuma powder

2 teaspoons chaga mycelium powder

1 teaspoon reishi mycelium powder

2 tablespoons cacao butter

2 tablespoons coconut oil

1 to 3 tablespoons wild honey, maple syrup,
    birch syrup, or xylitol (optional)

Pour the hot, strained tea into your blender containing all the above ingredients and immediately blend. To get a clear liquid, be sure to pour the tea through a strainer into the blender. Blend well and serve warm.

This is a wonderful drink to share with friends on a cold winter evening.

Serves: 3 to 4

Chaga as Food

Wild chaga mushroom can be dried and ground down (preferably with a mortar and pestle) into a powder that can be used like flour in your food. My experience with chaga flour is that it is bioavailable and does digest completely. Some people argue this point, yet they, in almost every case, have never actually eaten raw, dried chaga powder (flour) in significant amounts over years of time.

Commercial chaga mycelium powder, as well as most other mushroom mycelium powders, are "ready-to-go" forms of flour.

Chagalagadingdongs

3 tablespoons cacao powder

2 heaping tablespoons cacao butter

2 tablespoons almond or cashew butter

1 tablespoon raw wild chaga powder

1 tablespoon chaga mycelium

1 tablespoon reishi mycelium

1 tablespoon maca

1 tablespoon wild honey, maple syrup, birch syrup, or xylitol

First, melt the cacao butter—a double-boiler system is recommended. Fill a pot halfway with water and then place a heat-resistant Mason glass jar or Pyrex container filled with two heaping tablespoons of cacao butter inside the pot of water. Heat the pot up and wait for the cacao butter to melt. Then pour the liquid cacao butter into a nice large mixing bowl with all the other ingredients. Mix thoroughly with a wooden spoon. Roll into balls, put on a plate, and put in the freezer. This potent recipe is rich.

Serves: 3 to 4

Wild Chaga Cherry Torte

8 tablespoons cacao powder

5 tablespoons cacao butter

5 tablespoons almond or cashew butter

5 tablespoons raw wild chaga powder

1 tablespoon lucuma

1 tablespoon mesquite

1 tablespoon maca

5 tablespoons wild cherry dust
   (see note at end of recipe)

4 to 7 tablespoons chaga mycelium powder

4 tablespoons bee pollen

3 tablespoons wild honey

1 tablespoon xylitol powder (birch-derived)

2 tablespoons tocotrienols

1 teaspoon vanilla powder

2 pinches sea salt

Mix honey, tocotrienols, birch xylitol, and vanilla in their own bowl until thoroughly amalgamated. Tocotrienols are also called "rice bran solubles." They provide a more complete array of vitamin E compounds and add depth to the flavor, texture, and sweetness of superfood/superherb recipes, including this one!

In another bowl, thoroughly mix the cacao, liquified cacao butter (use a double-boiler system), almond/cacao butter, wild chaga powder, lucuma, mesquite, maca, bee pollen, wild cherry dust, chaga mycelium, and sea salt.

Mix the sweeteners (honey, tocos, xylitol, and vanilla) in with the main ingredients. Thoroughly mix and pour into a nonaluminum pie frame or shallow Pyrex pan. Place in the freezer. When nearly frozen, slice and serve in small torte samples. This is an extraordinary dessert. We often modify this at home to include more wild foods (which we add after drying and powdering them).

Serves: 5 to 6

Special Note: Wild cherry dust is made by crushing dried wild cherries with a large granite mortar and pestle until the pits are cracked and powdered (as well as the fruits), then filtering the leftovers through a stainless-steel mesh strainer. The dust that falls through is the wild cherry dust. It contains bits of the pits and dried fruit and ideally very little shell. Some people are sensitive to the toxic aspects of cherries and should not use wild cherry dust.

Chaga as a Broth

Instead of water, you can use a light chaga-tea base to cook rice, quinoa, millet, amaranth, barley, etc. Cook as normal, and the grain will soak up the goodness of chaga, turning your meal into medicine! In the same way, use a light chaga tea as a broth base for your soups.

Berry Chaga Breakfast

2 to 3 cups mixed fresh berries
(should be primarily fresh blueberries and
secondarily raspberries, then blackberries,
Saskatoon berries, elderberries, gooseberries,
spikenard berries, etc.)

3 to 4 tablespoons organic cold-pressed,
extra virgin olive oil

1 heaping tablespoon raw organic honey

2 to 3 droppers full of chaga tincture

1 tablespoon chaga mycelium powder

Mix in a bowl with a spoon and serve.

Serves: 1 or 2

Chaga Chips

Pieces of chaga, especially the black bits, can be dehy-
drated to a crisp. These chaga chips make for delicious
healthy snacks for children and adults. They are hard,
but your teeth will still crunch them—these are not
recommended for people with damaged teeth. There is
a natural sweetness to these chaga chips, but if you'd
like them slightly sweeter, dry the black bits, candy
them in honey, then dehydrate them again.

The Maine Man Creamy Choco-Chaga Kefir
(Recipe by Chef Frank Giglio)

16 ounces cultured milk kefir

2 to 3 tablespoons raw cream

6 to 8 chaga capsules (empty contents) or bulk chaga powder (6 capsules = 1 tablespoon)

1/2 teaspoon pine pollen

3/4 cup frozen wild blueberries

1 teaspoon vanilla powder

2 tablespoons cacao nibs

1 pinch sea salt

A touch of honey, maple syrup, stevia, or xylitol

For instructions on how to create nut- and seed-mylk kefirs (for use in place of the cultured milk kefir above), please see page 90.

Blend the entire recipe for 30 to 45 seconds in a high-speed blender. This is a great creamy super-nutrition probiotic milkshake treat for the entire family.

Serves: 3 to 4

Chaga, Philosopher-King

Amongst the tulle mists
That wander in gists
And twirl
Through leafless
Forests
Hyperborean swirls.
    A magical realm is near
Off fluttering fairy roads
Near cold springs, moss, toads
Hidden in fallen leaves,
Branches of trees,
A sum
Of running mycelium.
    Cosmic myco-spore journey through the eons
Fallen to Earth: ocean, ground,
To dwell secretly without a sound
Until the moment
When life factors ferment,
Forming every kind of nutriment.
Then they assist.
Gathering, enlist. . .
Making nutrients available by:
Swim, dig, fly.
Building life for life

Chaga

In a greater richness and diversity,
A superterranean university.
Soon growth, increase,
Spiral motions—without cease.
Across the land stretch shade and moisture.
The 'scape comes alive, filled with . . .
Bark, leaves, twigs, shells, nuts, pith
Mushroom caps, insects, ponds
Zen event horizons
Myco-relationship tips
Built upon relationship flop flips
Until at last . . . a forest.
Then, boreal density,
Intensity.
    Those myco-denizens of soil
That evolved into arboreal toil
To concentrate
Minerals that levitate
And ascend
In cycles without end
To outer space again.
    The light of you—polypore
Nestled in lore
Noble archetypes in chitin, wood
Medicines shamans understood.
Your spore release
In a moment cease,
Ormus from Earth's crust

Blown in poofs of dust.
 Of these . . .
A polypore spore
And one more
A symbiont extremophile
Unique in look, feel, style
Align lignin wind
And take wing
To take the throne as King.
 King of the Mushrooms: Chaga
Your role, critical in the Saga
In the Earth's fate
And unfolding drama.
Philosopher, teacher
Ally, healer.
In hallowed forests the fairies sing:
"All hail the Philosopher-King!"
 In royal pageantry
Bursting from the tree
Phallic, stellar
A touch of color
Orange, brown, black, charred
Betulinic, inspired.
 Mammoth medicine lost
Found by shaman's past
In search of the creative:
The posological native
Chaga hunter, eyes starred, wide,

Chaga

The touch of an enchanted side
Imbibed, felt, spied
And each new one tried,
Its own cosmic ride.
Alkaloids stimulate.
Thoughts abate.
A creative, timeless state.
    King commands jesters,
The testers:
Amanitas: *muscaria, pantherinas*
Partners with Queen
Elusive, exclusive
Red reishi unseen.
Commands from birch towers
Unleashing taiga powers
The tea, the brew
Lupeol stew
Maple-rich color
Hints vanilla flavor
Wood-burning
Spring water savior
Imagine you ingested
A perennial mirror, inflected
Upon which the cosmos is reflected.
Heals the thick
Youthens the bold
Drives the idea-pill
Into forests chill.

Sculptor of royal beauty
Classic *hauteur*.
Chiseled
With eyes that look past and through.
In the present,
Brand new.
Untouched by years
Nourished by snow, rain (never tears)
Never more needed
Completely undefeated.
    Chaga brings strength of righteousness,
Heaven smiles upon its growth,
Yes. Consecrated.
Fated.
    Lives endophytic in soil, tree
To rise to see
The celestial sea
One day bursting, emerging
To live upon the solar pour,
Heliovore, galactovore.
Chlorophyll an ally, sure
Within melanin
Pigments store
Energy for
The Great Work.
    Ideal birch forests, trees
Minus forty degrees
Circumpolar region extremes

Chaga

Where chaga commands scenes
Benevolent
Heaven scent.
Divine right
Cosmonaut enlight
Dreaming another cosmic endeavor
Planning The Best Future Ever.

— DAVID WOLFE
AVALON, ONTARIO, CANADA
© DECEMBER 2011

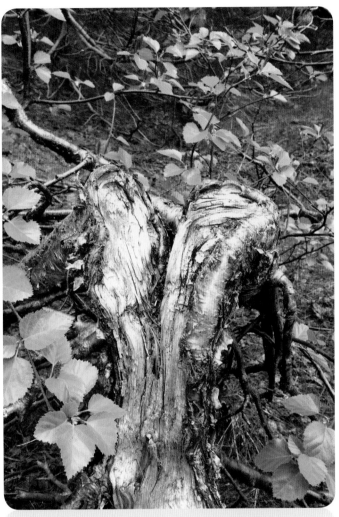

Under extraordinary Arctic conditions, chaga's host tree birch can survive and thrive.

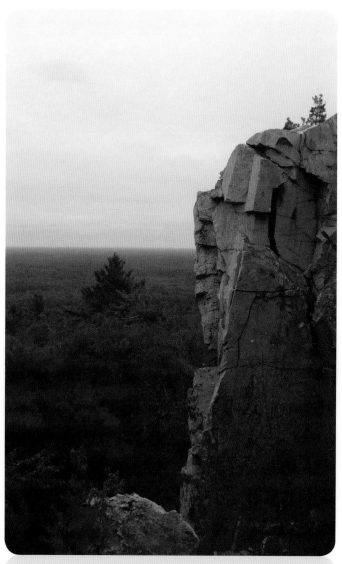

Chaga shamanic realms

Part III
The Science on Chaga

This portion of the book provides an in-depth look at how chaga delivers its magic. Please refer to the cited studies and the listed Internet sources for additional research. The exploration of chaga by science is far from complete, and we are likely to learn much more in the future about this amazing superherb.

Betulin, Betulinic Acid, and the Healing Properties of Birch

The promising medicinal properties of triterpene compounds that are particularly concentrated in chaga and reishi mushrooms continue to be uncovered by science. Healing effects range from fighting cancer to improving digestion, from lowering harmful LDL cholesterol to detoxifying the liver, from fighting viruses to alleviating asthma. Of the triterpenes, betulin and its metabolites betulinic acid and lupeol appear to be the most powerful and possess the broadest health benefits.

Present in the bark of all birch tree types, betulin is the white shiny powdery material that is most easily identified in the bark of white birch. Betulin concentrations vary among different types of birch trees and even vary widely among the same type of birch. For example, levels of betulin in the outer bark of four species of white-barked birch ranged from 5% to 22% in one study.[1] Birch bark can contain up to 35% betulin by dry-matter weight.[2] Betulin may also be found in other plants such as the great Ayurvedic brain-enhancing superherb *Bacopa monnieri*.

White-birch bark remains white, even when the tree wood itself has completely rotted. The stability of the bark in wild Nature is attributed to the antimicrobial properties of betulin and its related compounds.

John Pezzuto of the University of Chicago is quoted on several chaga websites as stating "the activity of betulinic acid is one of the most promising discoveries amongst 2,500 plant extracts studied."[3] His work with betulin has been cited by cancer researcher Dr. Ralph Moss in his "Moss Reports."[4] In the presence of healthy cells, betulin is extremely safe—megadoses (600 mg/kg body weight) of triterpenes such as betulin are well tolerated.[5]

Betulin and betulinic acid, as well as the related compound lupeol, are lupane-type pentacyclic triterpenes that are created in birch bark and then further concentrated by chaga mushroom, which absorbs them from the birch bark and converts them into forms more easily ingested by humans. According to research cited in Paul Stamets's landmark book *Mycelium Running* (i.e., Kahlos et al.),[6] these powerful anticancer compounds are more heavily concentrated in the charcoal-like skin of wild chaga sclerotium, which contains 30% betulin. Fungal lanostanes (another type of triterpene) dominate the yellow-orange inner part of wild chaga. Even though lanostanes exhibit strong cytotoxicity toward carcinoma cells, their stronger suit is their antibacterial and anticandida properties.

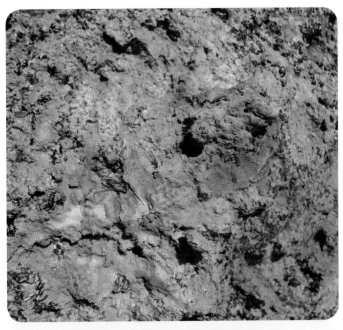

Wild chaga's foam core concentrates the lanostane triterpenoids.

Recent studies have shown that betulin, betulinic acid, and lupeol possess a wide spectrum of valuable pharmacological properties, including the following:

Anthelmintic. This is an herbal quality that expels parasitic worms.

Antibacterial. These triterpenes have been shown in vitro to eliminate the pathogens typhoid fever, tuberculosis, and diphtheria in three to ten minutes.

Anticancer. A wide variety of cancers have been studied using betulin and related compounds. One study reviewed the in vitro sensitivity to betulinic acid of broad cell-line panels derived from lung, colorectal, breast, prostate, and cervical cancer (which are the prevalent cancer types with the highest mortalities in women and men). The remarkable result: ". . . in all cell lines tested colony formation was completely halted at remarkably equal betulinic acid concentrations that are likely attainable in vivo. Our results substantiate the possible application of betulinic acid as a chemotherapeutic agent for the most prevalent human cancer types."[7] Chaga's low-pH betulinic acid apparently targets cancer cells because they also have a low pH (they are acidic).

Antihypoxant. Betulin decreases hypoxia (inadequate oxygen supply to the body's tissues) and increases the stability of the organism to an oxygen deficiency, thus helping to correct the metabolism of oxygen-deficient cells (e.g., cancer cells and virally contaminated cells).

Anti-inflammatory. As we age, the inflammatory response increases, possibly due to increasing levels of infection. Betulin and its related compounds fight infection, thereby reducing inflammation, thus helping us to become younger.

Antimalarial. Even though malaria is an infectious tropical disease, the temperate birch tree provides a strong antidote and medicine to its pernicious effects.[8]

Antimutagenic. Such a substance is capable of lowering the number of ongoing mutations in the chromosomes and genes that occur due to exposure to carcinogens, mutagens, and viruses. This action is connected with the capability of betulin and its metabolites to induce the production of interferons, which are well known to positively influence the processes of reparation of DNA.

Antioxidant. Peroxide free radicals are squelched by betulin and its related compounds, just like water being poured on fire.

Antiseptic. Not only does the birch bark possess antiseptic qualities, but it has also been traditionally used to make antiseptic-activated charcoal. Activated charcoals are known to neutralize some poisons and treat stomachaches, and they are still commonly used today.

Antitumor. Betulinic acid has selective cytotoxicity against melanoma, neuroectodermal, and malignant brain tumor cell lines;[9] it has been found to be active against other tumor types as well. Research on mice

indicates that betulinic acid is naturally attracted to sites
in the body where tumors are present.[10] This strong antitumor activity comes with virtually no side effects and
no toxicity. Betulinic acid works selectively on tumor
cells to cause apoptosis (spontaneous cell disassembly/
death), possibly because the interior pH of tumor tissues is generally lower than that of normal tissues, and
betulinic acid is only active at those lower levels.

Antipyretic. Betulinic acid reduces or quells fevers.

Antiviral. These compounds are currently being
tested for effectiveness in treating HIV/AIDS, several
different types of herpes,[11] and respiratory syncytial
virus (RSV, which can cause severe coldlike symptoms
and pneumonia).

Bile-expelling. Betulinic acid improves the secretion
of bile from the gallbladder, thus improving liver function, increasing digestive capacity, and protecting the
gallbladder.

Immunomodulatory. Betulinic acid induces the activation of macrophage and proinflammatory cytokines.
This appears to provide a molecular basis for the ability
of betulinic acid to mediate macrophage activity, suppress
inflammation, and modulate the immune response.[12]

Infection-fighting. Topically applied betulin has
been shown to help wounds heal more rapidly. Ancient
Russian medical manuals recommend birch for treating purulent wounds: "so that the rotten meat from

the ulcer was eaten away, ground birch crust should be poured into the rotten wound."[13]

Skin-protective. Skin care and cosmetic companies have begun adding birch bark extract to various products. Betulin and its related compounds betulinic acid and lupeol fight topical infections and irritations while simultaneously stimulating the growth of healthy skin cells.

How Beta Glucans Help Us Heal

Of all the compounds contained in chaga mushroom, perhaps the most well-studied is a type of polysaccharide known as "beta glucans." Today more than a thousand modern research studies have been conducted into the use and treatment of disease with beta glucans.

The capacity of the innate immune system to quickly recognize and respond to invading pathogens, viruses, harmful bacteria, free-radical (radiation) damage, and other potentially harmful environmental toxins is essential for all life forms to maintain homeostasis. The immune response–potentiating effect of beta glucans has been found in all branches of the animal, bird, fish, and plant kingdoms.

Within our bodies, beta glucans are bioactive molecules that act as potent "biological response modulators," activating the immune system. Beta glucans are the key activator in the process of phagocytosis, whereby white macrophage blood cells engulf and destroy harmful and diseased foreign substances in the body. Beta glucans have also been shown to stimulate various other immune effector cells, including B, NK, and T-cells, increasing the production of immunomodulating cytokines (interleukin 1 and interleukin 2) and antibodies. Beta glucans also potentiate the activities of various immune mediators, including lymphokines, which trigger more white blood cell production and activity and are thus an important component in the immune response.

One of the main reasons that beta glucans have become a subject of increased scientific focus is their consistent and direct connection to dramatically speeding the recovery from, reducing, and in many cases completely removing free-radical/radiation-damaged (cancerous) tissues and cellular debris. "Beta glucans

White Blood Cells

neutrophil   eosinophil   basophil   monocyte   lymphocyte

© apple1/Shutterstock.com

Different types of white blood cells

is proven to be effective at inhibiting mutagenic and immunomodulating effects of cancerous tumors by triggering various immune system responses."[14]

Rather than the introduction of toxic chemotherapy and isolated pharmaceutical compounds used in many cancer treatments that kill both healthy and "sick" cells, beta glucans simply stimulate and nourish naturally occurring immune cells, which are then able to selectively recognize and destroy mutated/sick cells.

Chemically speaking, beta glucans consist of a structure composed of repeating units of D-glucose molecules, and they come in a large variety of nonlinear shapes and molecular weights.

All beta glucans are linked by a 1,3 linear beta glycosidic chain core, and they differ from each other by their length and branching structures. The branches derived from the glycosidic chain core are highly variable, and the two main groups of branches are 1,4 and 1,6 glycosidic chains. These branching assignments appear to be species-specific; for example, beta glucans of mushrooms such as chaga have 1,6 side branches, whereas those of bacteria have 1,4 side branches. The alignments of branching follow a particular ratio, and branches can arise from branches (forming secondary branches).

It has been suggested that a higher degree of polysaccharide and glucans complexity (as demonstrated in chaga and all medicinal mushrooms) is associated with more potent immunomodulatory and anticancer effects.

Some key well-studied chaga polysaccharides include beta (1,3) (1,6) glucans and alpha (1,3) glucans. The word "beta" signifies the unique fashion in which the glucose molecules are formed together (as opposed to "alpha").

Research evidence indicates that glucans molecules work best to facilitate healing in synergy with other polysaccharides, triterpenes, sterols, and antioxidants (all of which are contained in chaga). Once again,

The Power of Beta Glucans

The following conditions respond favorably to beta glucans:[15]

Abdominal adhesions	Coronary artery disease
Abdominal sepsis	Dermatitis
Acute renal failure	Diabetes
Allergies	*E. coli* infection
Anthrax poisoning	Exercise stress
Autoimmune disorders	Fibromyalgia
Cancer	Free-radical damage
Candida albicans	Fungal disease
Carcinoma	Heart disease
Chromoblastomycosis	Hepatitis
Chronic fatigue syndrome	Herpes (all types)
Cold sores (herpes)	High LDL Cholesterol
Colorectal surgery	Leprosy

scientists are confirming that any single molecule or compound never acts ideally alone, but rather the sum of all parts works intelligently and harmoniously to form a complex "living medicine."

Chaga's beta glucans are known to have antibacterial, anti-inflammatory, antiallergenic, liver-protective, anti-tumor, immune amphoteric (for reducing blood pressure), and anticarcinogenic properties, to name a few. Extractions of these polysaccharide compounds from

(... continued from the previous page)

Leucopenia	Peritonitis
Leukemia	Pneumonia
Lipid metabolism disorder	Rabies
Liver damage	Radiation damage
Low platelet production	Rheumatoid arthritis
Lung damage	Sarcoma
Lupus	Skin regeneration
Malaria	Spinal cord injury
Melanoma	Staph infection
Microbial infection	Stem-cell transplant
Multiple sclerosis	Trauma recovery
Mycotoxins	Tuberculosis
Oxidation damage	Ulcers
Parasites	Wound healing
	Viral infections

the chaga mushroom have also been shown to have strong antimutagenic and antioxidative effects that inhibit genotoxicity, or the mutation and formation of tumors from otherwise healthy cells.[16]

The Essential Role of Macrophages in the Immune System

Beta glucans are the most widely and commonly observed natural activators of the Earth's most ancient and immunologically competent immune cell—the macrophage. Macrophages are found not only in humans, higher animals, and vertebrates, but they are also found in primitive invertebrates such as the hydra, which has no other immunological cells, only macrophages. There are literally billions of macrophages found in all the tissues, organs, blood, and lymph of the human body!

The macrophage is a critical part of the immune system, as it is the "intelligence" which represents the first line of defense in the initiation and maintenance of the immune response. Macrophages are scientifically classified as phagocytes. These large white blood cells are responsible for finding, identifying, breaking down, and removing foreign particles and pathogens such as bacteria, yeast cells, tumor cells, and virally infected cells in the body (a process called phagocytosis).

Originating in the bone marrow from a pluripotent stem cell, each new macrophage enters the blood stream as a monocyte, where it then matures and activates into its final stage and enters into the tissues as part of the human body's defense force. Through its growth cycle a sequence of metabolic changes occurs, resulting in the stimulated production of essential immune-supporting substances, including cytokines such as interleukin 1. These cytokines stimulate the overall immune system and boost bone marrow production.

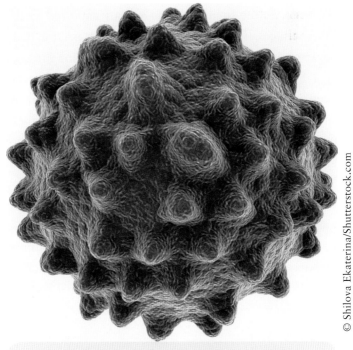

The white blood cell protects and serves.

Beta glucans act as keys that turn on the body's macrophage defense response, beginning with the increased production of stem cells[17] in the bone marrow[18] and then cascading into events that "supercharge" the macrophages as they develop. These white blood cells mature and then devour and remove antigens, pathogens, toxins, and cellular waste debris.

Specifically, here is how it works: the beta glucans found in chaga, other herbs, foods, or supplements enter the body via the small intestine and are captured by the macrophages. To be activated by beta glucans, the macrophages must first "ingest" the beta glucans through specific beta glucan receptor sites on these cells' membranes. Then the macrophages internalize and fragment the beta glucans within themselves and transport these fragments to the bone marrow (helping stimulate more stem cells) and to the reticuloendothelial system (RES). The beta glucans fragments are eventually released by the macrophages and taken up by other immune cells, including neutrophils, monocytes, natural killer cells, and dendritic cells, leading to numerous enhanced immune responses,[19] including adaptability against and deactivation of foreign pathogens, genotoxicity (toxins harmful to genetics), cancerous growth formations, and environmental toxicity.

According to a study that appeared in the *Journal of Hematology and Oconology* in 2009, "animals pretreated with purified glucan particles are subsequently more resistant to bacterial, viral, fungal, and protozoan challenge, reject antigenically incompatible grafts more rapidly and produce higher titers of serum antibodies to specific antigens."[20]

The Antioxidative Power of Beta Glucans

The existence of cancer and other tumors within the body is extremely stressful and can create large amounts of free-radical damage. As the immune system begins to adapt to the influx of beta glucans and the other chemical constituents of chaga, one of the first things to subside within the body is the oxidative damage and stress caused by free radicals.

Even oxidative damage caused and induced by external injury from burns and other means can be effectively treated by both local and systemic administration of beta glucans.[21] Their wide-ranging antioxidant properties have (intriguingly) been shown to "mediate [even] its radioprotection by enhancing resistance to microbial invasion mechanism[s] not necessarily predicated on hemopoietic [formation of blood cells] recovery," meaning that as macrophages activate themselves in an oxidized environment, they "have been shown to selectively phagocytize [ingest] and sequester glucan," suggesting that "these specific cells may be protected by virtue of glucan's scavenging abilty."[22]

Skin-Regenerative Effects of Beta Glucans and Chaga

Because of high commercial and cultural interest, a great deal of research is currently underway to determine the capability of beta glucans to "youthen" and heal skin. Consider the following report from one such study:

"The effect of a cosmetic regimen containing beta-1,3-glucan on the signs of aging in the skin was evaluated in 150 women, ages 35 to 60. A 27 percent improvement in skin hydration was observed after eight weeks of using the regimen twice a day. A measurable improvement in lines and wrinkles at the end of the study reached 47 percent, firmness and elasticity increased by 60 percent, and skin color improved by 26 percent."[23]

In addition, evidence indicates that beta glucans protect the skin from burns when applied topically and also when taken internally.[24]

As is explored in the next section, chaga has a particular affinity for fighting melanomas (skin cancer), and evidence indicates that beta glucans plays a role in this skin-protective effect, as does melanin. Chaga's affinity for the skin indicates that skin diseases such as psoriasis should respond favorably to ingesting chaga tea, which has been noted in the scientific literature.[25]

Chaga's Melanin Content

Melanin (Greek μέλας, meaning "black") is a pigment found throughout the natural world. It has been detected in most organisms (with the exception of spiders, and the prevalence of melanin in the Archaea and Bacteria kingdoms is an issue of ongoing scientific debate). A form of melanin makes up the ink used by the octopus and other cephalopods as a shield against danger. Melanin is what gives wild chaga its distinctive coloration, and it also creates color in human skin.

Melanins are constructed of electrically conductive polymers: polyacetylene, polypyrrole, and polyaniline. Various proportions and bonding angles of these different polymers create different types of melanin. Dopamelanin, eumelanin (a brown-black polymer), and pheomelanin (a red-brown polymer responsible for red hair and freckles) are common types of melanin pigments. Eumelanin is a dominant melanin in humans; the white appearance of an albino is largely a result of a deficiency of this pigment.

Chaga contains more melanin than any other food or herb known; it is the best nutritional source of the compound, containing pigments similar to those found in the human body. Chaga's melanin demonstrates high antioxidant and genoprotective effects.[26]

In humans, melanin is found in:

Skin: Melanin is a primary determining factor in one's skin color. It is produced by melanocytes found in the basal layer of the epidermis. Even though all humans contain about the same amount of melanocytes in their skin, the melanocytes in some people and different ethnic groups produce differing amounts of melanin, thereby resulting in differing skin colors and qualities.

Hair: Melanin in the hair provides its color.

Iris: The color of one's iris is indicated by the eye's concentration of melanin.

Inner ear (stria vascularis): Those with more melanin production (darker skin and eye pigments) may be less susceptible to inner-ear damage and hearing loss.[27]

Nervous system: Pigment-bearing neurons throughout the nervous system contain melanin, including areas of the brainstem (such as the medulla, locus coeruleus, and the substantia nigra). Melanin is also found in the zona reticularis of the adrenal glands. Corticotropin, the pituitary hormone that stimulates the adrenals, alters melanin production throughout the body.

Pineal gland: According to researcher and friend David Wilcock, who is likely the world's leading expert on activating the pineal gland, the pineal gland requires melanin in order to function optimally. In fact, says Wilcock, the pineal gland requires melanin more than any other nutrient.[28]

Melanin is a nutritionally demanding pigment; this means that to create melanin, strong nutrient demands are put on the body. Oftentimes with age, stress, genetic triggers, and mineral-deficient nutrition, melanin formation in the skin may be disturbed, causing white spots and possibly leading to vitiligo (which appears to be stress-related and may have viral components).[29] Having a nutritional source of melanin such as chaga lightens the body's load of nutrient-demanding processes involved in melanogenesis (the formation of melanin).

Melanin, as a nutrient, enhances the beauty and appearance of one's hair, skin, and eyes. It helps to restore and maintain a more youthful appearance. Melanin functions as a neurologically active protein (that is, a neuropeptide, found concentrated in the neurons that produce important neurotransmitters such as serotonin, dopamine, and adrenalin. Ingesting melanin in the diet (in the form of chaga) may have health-giving effects on all the body parts listed above.

Melanin pigments interact with all types of radiation: light, heat, and kinetic energy. Some types of fungi, called radiotrophic fungi, appear to be able to use melanin as a photosynthetic pigment that enables them to capture gamma rays and harness its energy for growth.[29a] Melanin compounds found in many organisms, including chaga and the human body, possess photoprotectant qualities: they absorb harmful UV radiation frequencies and convert them to harmless heat through a process termed "ultrafast internal conversion." This process allows the melanin to dissipate an estimated 99.9% of the absorbed UV radiation as heat. Because of this, melanin compounds are able to protect all types of organisms, including bacteria and fungi, against the stresses of solar UV radiation and aggressive free radicals. In humans, ultrafast internal conversion and the natural increased production of melanin (melanogenesis) help create a tan, yet also prevent the cumulative, indirect DNA damage induced by UV (B-type) radiation that eventually leads to the development of various skin cancers, including malignant melanoma.

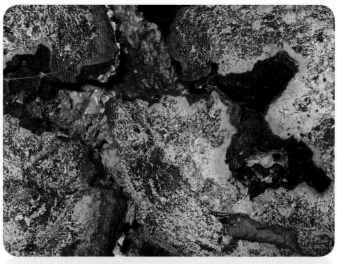

Chaga's interior pigments

It appears that chaga's effects on healing human skin cancers have something to do with its melanin content, which nutritionally enables more ultrafast internal conversion. In the same way, chaga's melanin compounds are able to help deactivate radioactive isotopes, converting them into benign forms. This may be the primary reason why wild chaga is protective against radiation treatments (including types of chemotherapy) and radioactive fallout (e.g., Fukushima). But note that chaga mycelium products (grown in the controlled environment) have never been shown to possess the radioprotective properties that wild chaga possesses (although future innovations in mycelium-growing technologies may change this).

Melanin also protects many organisms, including humans, against cellular damage due to high temperatures, chemical stresses (such as heavy metals), and biochemical attack threats, because it improves immunological defenses against pathogens.

Putting it all together, we can conclude that the human frame may be aided by taking chaga products, because their melanin content influences, protects, and aids one's hearing, pineal gland, adrenals, nervous system, skin, immune system, and genetics. Melanin's DNA-protective action and its influence on the nervous system make it one of the most important biological compounds for maintaining mental health and even developing deeper levels of consciousness and intelligence.

Chaga vs. Cancer:
Let the Science Talk

Contributed by Pierre Beaumier and Ramiz Saad[30]

The following section contains exciting up-to-date laboratory data, recently compiled by my associates studying the biological constituents of chaga.—David Wolfe

A cornucopia of compounds and components make up chaga's impressive medicinal character, including betulin, betulinic acid, triterpenes, sterols, a high concentration of superoxide dismutase (SOD), polysaccharides, beta glucans, melanin, and many minerals. Chaga has a rich concentration of sterols and other compounds that are synthesized and extracted from the birch tree that the mushroom lives on. Some of the specific triterpenes and sterols that have medicinal properties are lanosterol, ergosterol (a precursor to vitamin D), and inotodiol, all of which are in alcohol extracts of chaga. In vivo research using the ethanol extract showed a growth-inhibitory rate (74.6%) of cancer cells.[31]

This section focuses on an aspect of the chaga that has yet to be discussed to any extent in the scientific literature: the aqueous and alcohol extracts of chaga, which exhibit significant antitumor activity.[32] The inorganic components (minerals) will be discussed here, as opposed to the organic fraction, which contains all of the healing components just mentioned.

A good deal of effort has been expended trying to grow chaga in the laboratory, since the natural reserves of the mushroom are limited. Wild chaga is the most potent source of medicinal compounds, yet a comparison of the potency of extracts from wild chaga, cultivated chaga, and cultivated fruiting body reveals the following percentages: 86.1%, 59.9%, and 71.8%, respectively.[33] Thus, although wild chaga is the most powerful, cultivated chaga shows good activity too.

In a recent study, the antioxidant activity of a hot-water extract of chaga was precisely compared with those of other medicinal fungi *(Agaricus blazei, Mycelia, Ganoderma lucidum,* and *Phellinus linteus).* Chaga showed the strongest antioxidant activity among fungi examined, in terms of both superoxide and hydroxyl radicals' scavenging activities.[34]

We studied the water extracts and alcohol extracts using an ICPMS-DRC, which is the latest in instrumentation for studying/examining minerals in biological specimens. This instrument allows researchers to look at levels of minerals in parts per trillion, which has not been done in the past.

It is our opinion that aqueous and alcohol extracts of chaga have medicinal properties based not only on soluble organic compounds, but also on the high concentrations of cesium (Cs+), rubidium (Rb+), and potassium (K+) present in chaga. If chaga is king of the mushrooms, we can call these three components the king, queen, and prince of alkaline elements. All are water-soluble and easily extracted from chaga into aqueous media. Chaga can undergo multiple extractions, with the first being the most concentrated, as seen in the figure below.

The data were generated by placing the chaga sample in a teapot with water that was brought to a boil. Then the heat was reduced, and the chaga was allowed to simmer for 10 minutes. The process was repeated four times, using the same chaga and equal amounts of water. Rubidium (same profile for cesium or potassium) was still being extracted in the fourth extraction. An alkaline pH of 9.6 was observed for the first water extracts. Rubidium, cesium, and potassium are among the most alkaline elements in nature. They are also present in alcohol extracts of chaga (available

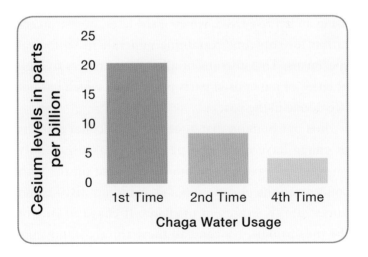

commercially), as the alcohol extracts are 40% alcohol and 60% water.

The quantities of cesium, rubidium, and potassium in chaga by far exceed the levels found in any other food source. The only other sources with high levels of all three are green tea and orange pekoe tea. In the table below, the results of laboratory analysis show that those two teas are good, but chaga tea is the best—and does not contain caffeine.

Element*	Chaga	Green Tea	Orange Pekoe Tea
Cesium	.72	.42	.34
Rubidium	490	41	31
Potassium	149,411	15,830	13,627

*All measurements are in parts per million.

The Hopi Indians in Arizona have a very low cancer rate (1 in 1000) compared to the rest of the United States (1 in 4). Their diet has been shown to have very high levels of rubidium and potassium compared to the average American diet.[35] In addition, areas in North and South America where the soil is volcanic show higher-than-normal levels of cesium, rubidium, and potassium, and correspondingly lower cancer rates. Hawaii has lower cancer rates (4.3%) than the rest of the United States (5% to 9%), and this relationship of volcanic soil and lower cancer rates is also found in areas of Peru and Ecuador. Lower cancer rates probably contribute to the longer life expectancy in Hawaii: 79.8 years compared to 76.9 years for the rest of the country. Hawaii also has the best cancer-survival rate—10% higher than all other states.[36]

Again, the benefit of living in volcanic areas stems from the alkaline soil, which is rich in cesium, rubidium, and potassium. Because these elements are water-soluble, they would be elevated in the drinking water and would be readily absorbed by plants. It is important to realize that the elevated levels of the three elements we are discussing are caused by the concentrating effects of specific plants grown in these soils. Research suggests that mushrooms are very good at concentrating alkaline elements.[37] In some cases, this can be a negative for human consumption, such as when a high arsenic level in soil is concentrated by an edible mushroom.

In response to the Chernobyl disaster, a Swedish study looked at using the concentrating effect of mushrooms to monitor radioactive cesium following a nuclear explosion.[38] (Note that natural cesium, cesium-133, which we've been referring to, is not radioactive, but cesium-137 is radioactive and is formed during nuclear explosions.)

Many scientific papers highlight the anticancer effects of cesium based on the alkaline nature of the element.[39] In 1931, the Nobel Prize for Physiology or Medicine was given to Dr. Otto Warburg, who discovered that cancer cells go into self-destruct mode (apoptosis) in alkaline environments, and that in acidic environments, cancer cells proliferate.

In one study with fifty cancer patients—the majority considered terminal cases (advanced disease)—there was a 50% recovery rate from various cancers following a three-year cesium chloride treatment.[40] Most of those who died did so within a few weeks (26%) to one year (24%) after starting treatment. This study has been quoted many times but remains controversial, as few in the medical community have continued in this direction. Cesium chloride can be toxic at high concentrations, which may be one reason why no clinical trials based on this research have followed.

Two other elements that are important to the body's fight against cancer are germanium and zinc, both of which are involved with the immune system.

Germanium itself is not abundant in nature and is not found in any high concentrations in food. The germanium found in chaga would be considered "organic" germanium. The taking of germanium supplements has produced serious side effects (kidney problems); however, germanium obtained from plants tends to be water-insoluble and carries little toxicity. Some complex organic germanium compounds have been investigated as potential pharmaceutical agents. At this point none have reached the market.

Zinc's important role in the body involves hundreds of enzymes, as well as the immune system. It contributes to normal growth during adolescence and to our sense of taste and smell. The body does not store zinc, so we need a daily intake in order to function properly.

Levels of germanium and zinc elements in chaga are very high compared to other foods (see the chart below).

Food*	Germanium	Zinc
Chaga	0.44	370
Chocolate	0.06	51
Orange Pekoe Tea	0.02	29
Green Tea	0.08	38
Turmeric	0.04	18
Soy Beans	0.02	28
Walnuts	0.01	40
Chick Peas	0	32
Apple	0.01	<1
Banana	0.01	2
Turnip	0	2.5
Liver	0	42
Spinach	0	7
Olive Oil	0	<1
Shrimp	0	15
Asparagus	0	5
Carrot	0	2
Beef	0	22
Basmati Rice	0	17

*All measurements in parts per million

Chaga has a dark outer skin and a light-brown interior. Analysis showed the following elemental differences.

Element*	Outside Skin	Interior
Iron	28	40
Copper	20	10
Zinc	380	190
Germanium	n/a	n/a
Potassium	133,000	59,000
Rubidium	464	156
Cesium	1.7	3

*All measurements in parts per million

The composition of chaga can vary, depending on the country of origin, the soil's concentrations of the elements, the health of the chaga, and the season the chaga was harvested. To better understand the variations based on origin, chaga specimens from different countries around the world and from several regions of Canada were analyzed. The samples were obtained from chaga sellers and individuals who were contacted to obtain local chaga samples. One sample came from chaga growing on a fallen tree. Another sample was taken from a chaga fruit (that is, a new growth that the chaga forms as it tries to spread). A third sample, from the same area, was taken from chaga that seemed to have died and that was partially detached from the tree. The same tree had healthy chaga higher up on the tree. To understand where the chaga would get the cesium and rubidium from, samples of birch bark were also analyzed. The results are presented in the table on page 151.

"Ash percent" is the residue remaining after water and organic materials are removed by heating the sample. This number represents the minerals that were present in the sample. As seen in the table, the higher the ash content in the chaga, the more cesium, rubidium, and potassium—as well as other minerals—were present. The zinc and manganese levels in the birch bark are elevated; the chaga does not concentrate these elements but reflects what is normal on the tree bark. Note that the average concentration of rubidium seen in a number of other mushrooms is elevated.

It is very clear from the table that the quality of chaga differs greatly if we look only at the three key elements. The birch bark does have some cesium, rubidium, and potassium; however, chaga seems to be efficient at concentrating these elements. The chaga taken from a dead fallen tree still had good levels of rubidium and potassium, but the cesium had disappeared. It's possible that the level of cesium may be a measure of the health of the chaga. The dead chaga on the live tree showed depletion of the key elements, possibly due to dilution caused by rain.

Region	Ash %	Cesium	Rubidium	Potassium	Zinc	Manganese
Chaga fruit	4.9	0.08	19	1500	78	460
Canada AB	4.9	0.01	2.7	1500	95	23
Canada NB	10	0.16	77	37,000	75	340
Can. ON-1	13.5	0.42	190	47,500	110	190
Can. ON-2	12.7	0.72	490	149,000	210	320
Can. ON-3	10.7	0.47	175	42,600	90	230
Can. Dead tree chaga	6.31	0.06	80	24,000	130	210
Can. Live tree dead chaga	2.21	0.01	2.4	630	160	1000
USA	1.6	0.01	0.88	2,240	29	5
Siberia	10.46	0.16	78	49,400	42	260
Poland	5.5	0.57	64	26,300	40	190
White Birch Bark	1.1	0.02	1.07	350	110	630
Silver Birch Bark	0.86	0.01	0.4	160	76	420
Mushroom avg 12 types*	N/A	N/A	31	N/A	8.6	14.6

* From *The Finnish Environment* 25 (2008)

Let's not forget that there is fiber present in the mushroom, both soluble and insoluble types. Wikipedia defines these two fibers as:

- soluble (prebiotic, viscous): fiber that is readily fermented in the colon into gases and physiologically active byproducts
- insoluble: fiber that is metabolically inert, absorbing water as it moves through the digestive system, easing defecation

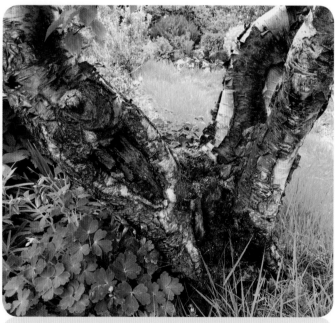

The extraordinary bark of Icelandic birch: *Betula pubescens*

The laboratory analysis of chaga shows that insoluble fiber is 61% of the mushroom's total weight, and soluble fiber 3.9%—both are considered high levels. Many people have reported more ease in defecation following use of the alcohol extract of chaga. To benefit from the insoluble fiber, one would need to take chaga powder orally.

Chaga was analyzed in our laboratories for various sugars and vitamins as well. No fructose, glucose, sucrose, maltose, or lactose was detected. Of the vitamins, only vitamin B_2 (also known as riboflavin) was detected, at 3.4mg per 100g. Chaga was also analyzed for different allergens and common toxins (fumonisin, aflatoxin, soy allergens, egg allergens, gluten allergens, total milk allergens), none of which were detected.

It is estimated there are 140,000 different mushrooms on Earth, with only 10% known. Chaga has been studied to some extent because of its recorded biological activity over the centuries. Given the rich storehouse of nutrients in well-known medicinal mushrooms, imagine what else is yet to be learned from these humble substances.

Wild Chaga:
Nutrition and Medicine

Wild chaga is known to contain the following nutrients and natural medicines:

Water-soluble polysaccharides
Alcohol-soluble polysaccharides
Protein-bound polysaccharides
Beta glucans (polysaccharide)
Lanostane triterpenoids
Betulin and betulinic acid
Ergosterol peroxides
Lanosterols (trametenolic acid)
Superoxide dismutase (SOD)
Inotodiols
Saponins (triterpenoid type)
Melanin
Trace minerals: antimony, barium, bismuth, boron, germanium, copper, manganese, strontium, zinc
Major minerals: calcium, cesium, iron, magnesium, phosphorus, potassium, rubidium, silicon
Vitamins B_2, B_3, D_2, K_1
Dietary fiber
Amino acids (typically lower than other edible and medicinal mushrooms, yet bearing a nearly complete essential amino acid profile with the exception of isoleucine)

Part IV
Resources

Recommended Websites

In addition to the sites listed here, check out the Wikipedia entries for chaga mushroom and for:

- Betulinic acid—Betulin and betulinic acid are up-and-coming nutrients to watch for in the fight against cancer. It's important to avail yourself of this information.
- Melanin—This entry includes fascinating details about one of the Earth's most interesting natural compounds!
- *Shennong Ben Cao Jing*—This was the first known herbalism book. It covers 365 herbs, including chaga.

www.aumstar.com—contains interesting research on mushrooms, mythology, and language.
www.earthbornwellness.com/chagause.htm
www.survivaltopics.com/survival/the-chaga-natures -medicinal-mushroom—a great chaga website
http://botit.botany.wisc.edu/toms_fungi/polypore.html —a wonderful website about tree mushrooms, also known as polypores
http://mushroomnutrition.com/inonotus-obliquus
www.primitiveways.com/Iceman.html—great information on Otzi the Iceman and his equipment

Books

Mycelium Running, by Paul Stamets

MycoMedicinals: An Informational Treatise on Mushrooms, by Paul Stamets

Indian Herbalogy of North America, by Alma R. Hutchens (National Library of Ottawa), pp. 77–80

The Cancer Ward, by Aleksandr Solzhenitsyn—An essential book for those interested in chaga's literary history.

The Book of the Damned, by Charles Fort—Contains interesting accounts of strange rains, nostoc (mushroom spores), animals, and objects falling from the sky.

The Source Field Investigations, by David Wilcock—Though mentioned in these pages for its discussion of the pineal gland, this book extensively covers many interesting subjects and is perhaps the best book on metaphysics ever written—a triumphant achievement. Savor every page.

Scientific Articles

General

Ron Spinosa, "The Chaga Story," *The Mycophile* (Journal of the North American Mycological Association) 47, no. 1 (January/February 2006): 1, 8, 23.

W. Zheng, K. Miao, Y. Liu, Y. Zhao, M. Zhang, S. Pan, et al., "Chemical diversity of biologically active metabolites in the sclerotia of *Inonotus obliquus* and submerged culture strategies for up-regulating their production," *Appl. Microbiol. Biotechnol.* 87, no. 4 (2010): 1237–54.

X. H. Zhong, K. Ren, S. J. Lu, S. Y. Yang, and D. Z. Sun, "Progress of research on *Inonotus obliquus*," *Chin. J. Integr. Med.* 15, no. 2 (April 2009): 156–60.

Antioxidant Properties

Yong Cui, Dong-Seok Kim, and Kyoung-Chan Park, "Antioxidant effect of *Inonotus obliquus*," *Journal of Ethnopharmacology* 96, nos. 1 and 2 (January 2005): 79–85.

Antiviral Properties

Ulrike Lindequist, Timo H. J. Niedermeyer, and Wolf-Dieter Jülich "The Pharmacological Potential of Mushrooms," *eCAM* 2, no. 3 (2005): 285–99.

Conclusions: This broad article on the immunological power of medicinal mushrooms includes discussion of chaga's potential to inhibit HIV protease and reishi's antiviral properties.

Anticancer Properties

J. Burczyk, A. Gawron, M. Slotwinska, B. Smietana, K. Terminska, "Antimitotic activity of aqueous extracts of *Inonotus obliquus*," *Journal of Ethnopharmacology* 121, no. 2 (January 21, 2009): 221–28.

Source: Department of Pharmacognosy, Silesian Medical Academy, Sosnowiec, Poland.

From the Abstract: "The cytotoxic effect of two aqueous extracts of *Inonotus obliquus* on human cervical uteri cancer cells (Hela S3) in vitro was evaluated. It was concluded that Inonotus extracts at a concentration of 10 micrograms/ml to 2000 micrograms/ml inhibited cancer cells growth."

M. J. Youn et al., "Potential anticancer properties of the water extract of *Inonotus* [corrected] *obliquus* by induction of apoptosis in melanoma B16-F10 cells," *Boll. Chim. Farm.* 135, no. 5 (May 1996): 306–9.

Aim of the study: "To examine the anti-proliferative effects of *Inonotus obliquus* extract on melanoma B16-F10 cells."

Conclusion: This study showed that the water extract of *Inonotus obliquus* mushroom exhibited a potential anticancer activity against B16-F10 melanoma cells in vitro and in vivo through the inhibition of proliferation and induction of differentiation and apoptosis of cancer cells.

W. Mazurkiewicz et al. (July/August 2010), "Separation of an aqueous extract *Inonotus obliquus* (Chaga). A novel look at the efficiency of its influence on proliferation of A549 human lung carcinoma cells," *Acta Pol. Pharm.* 67, no. 4: 397–406.

M. J. Youn et al., "Chaga mushroom *(Inonotus obliquus)* induces G0/G1 arrest and apoptosis in human hepatoma HepG2 cells," *World J Gastroenterol.* 14, no. 4 (January 28, 2008): 511–17.

Conclusion: "Chaga mushroom may provide a new therapeutic option, as a potential anticancer agent, in the treatment of hepatoma."

Yong Ook Kim et al., "Immuno-stimulating effect of the endo-polysaccharide produced by submerged culture of *Inonotus obliquus,*" *Life Sciences* 77, no. 19 (2005): 2438–56.

Yong Ook Kim et al., "Anti-cancer effect and structural characterization of endo-polysaccharide from cultivated mycelia of *Inonotus obliquus,*" *Life Sciences* 79, no. 1 (May 30, 2006): 72–80.

Antitumor Properties

K. Kahlos, L. Kangas, and R. Hiltunen, "Antitumor activity of some compounds and fractions from an n-hexane extract of *Inonotus obliquus* in vitro," *Acta Pharm. Fennica* 96 (1987): 33–40.

Melanin Content

J. Burczyk, A. Gawron, M. Slotwinska, B. Smietana, and K. Terminska, "Antimitotic activity of aqueous extracts of Inonotus obliquus," *Boll. Chim. Farm.,* 135 (1996): 306–9.

V. G. Babitskaya, V. V. Scherba, N. V. Ikonnikova, N. A. Bisko, and N. Y. Mitropolskaya, "Melanin complex from medicinal mushroom *Inonotus obliquus,*" *Int. J. Med. Mushrooms* 4 (2002): 139–45.

Chaga Products, Superherbs, and Superfoods

Explore your vast library of choices—what's in the cupboard of possibility? Today is the best day ever to experiment with raw and living foods, superfoods, and superherbs such as chaga: the "king of the mushrooms."

The following superfood and superherb products (and other unique products) are organically grown or wildcrafted and available now for your enjoyment at health-food stores and the online shop:

www.longevitywarehouse.com

Ant (Changbai mountain ant)

Ashwaganda

Asparagus root *(shatavari)*

Astragalus

Cacao beans

Cacao butter

Cacao nibs

Cacao powder

Camu berry powder

Cashews and cashew butter (products of extraordinary quality)

Cat's claw

Cayenne

Chaga (unique products including wild Canadian chaga)

Chanca piedra

Chlorella

Chocolate (Sacred Chocolate™, my personal line of raw chocolate products and exotic chocolates)

Coconut oil

Coconut cream (coconut butter)

Deer/Elk antler

Resources

E3 Live™ (blue-green
 algae)
Ginseng (world's leading
 selection of extracts)
Goji berries
Gynostemma (capsules,
 powders, and tea)
Hempseeds and their oil
Ho Shou Wu (Fo-Ti)
Honey (exclusive, rare
 NoniLand™ honey)
Horsetail (David Wolfe
 Bone Formula)
Incan berries
Kelp (and other seaweeds)
Maca (regular, red,
 black, etc.)

Maca Extreme
Mangosteen powder
Mucuna
Nettles (David Wolfe
 Bone Formula)
Noni
Marine phytoplankton
Olive oil (ice-pressed)
Pau d'arco
Reishi
Rhodiola
Schizandra berry
Shilajit
Spirulina
Tulsi
Vanilla

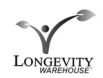

www.longevitywarehouse.com

Sacred Chocolate

Sacred Chocolate is clearly the best chocolate bar ever. Take one bite and you will know that Sacred Chocolate has cracked the cacao code!—David Wolfe

Sacred Chocolate™ is committed to bringing you the highest-quality chocolate ever. From the cacao bean to each chocolate bar, Sacred Chocolate is infused with love, prayer, and gratitude. We honor, respect, and give thanks to all beings that make possible the amazing superfood known as chocolate. *Theobroma cacao* is the scientific name for the chocolate tree, which means the "food of God." To our Sacred Chocolate team, this food is a holy sacrament, an offering to the higher power and a superfood for positive life transformation.

Our special chocolate is made over several days, the old-fashioned way: we slowly stone-grind raw cacao beans at a low temperature. Our cacao beans are never roasted, and all processes are kept below 114° Fahrenheit to ensure maximum antioxidant retention and zero trans-fatty acid production. Sacred Chocolate has an antioxidant rating (ORAC score) three to four

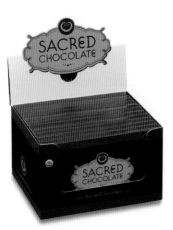

times higher than that of a cooked dark chocolate bar of comparable cacao content.

Our ingredients are raw (unroasted) wherever possible and always certified organic and/or wildcrafted. Sacred Chocolate is also certified vegan, kosher, and halal.

The Sacred Chocolate *Immuno Mushroom* chocolate bar is the only chocolate bar in the world that contains wild chaga.

Our cacao is sold above fair-trade standards. We never use weak cacao "filler" beans to boost the cacao percentages of our bars, and we completely avoid cane sugar in all our products. Sacred Chocolate comes in rectangular bars as well as in the shape of a heart to symbolize that raw chocolate is good for the heart and that great love and care go into the making of this superfood treat.

Sacred Chocolate is extremely low in caffeine and, like all chocolate, contains theobromine, which is greatly superior to caffeine, since theobromine has cardiovascular- and lung-healing properties. Theobromine does not affect the central nervous system or constrict blood vessels. For those who want to reduce their coffee consumption, Sacred Chocolate is the healthiest alternative. Theobromine dilates blood vessels and relaxes smooth muscle tissue, reducing the risk of cardiovascular challenges. For nearly four decades (1890–1930), theobromine was injected into the bloodstream to revive heart attack victims. Theobromine also relaxes bronchial muscles in the lungs. Studies indicate that theobromine acts on the vagus nerve, which runs from the lungs to the brain. For this reason, chocolate has been found to be effective in reducing asthma symptoms.

Sacred Chocolate is the only chocolate product in the world that includes the microbe-free skin of the cacao bean for flavor and nutritional purposes. The delicate skin adds a fruity complexity to the flavor of Sacred Chocolate and also contains concentrated phytonutrients, analogous to the nutrition found in the skin of most fruits and vegetables. Sacred Chocolate uses certified vegan, organic maple sugar in all sweetened recipes. The maple bouquet adds a rich complexity to the cacao bean. Also, by using maple, old-growth forests thrive— trees are not cut down to produce it. Maple rates low on the glycemic index with a score of fifty-five, and it contains manganese, zinc, and potassium, as well as antioxidants including epicatechins and quercetin.

A portion of Sacred Chocolate profits is donated to the Fruit Tree Planting Foundation (ftpf.org).

Now is the best time ever to visit www.SacredChocolate.com.

"Open the Heart . . . Discover the Magic!"

Peak Performance Archives: Enhance Your Health and Life

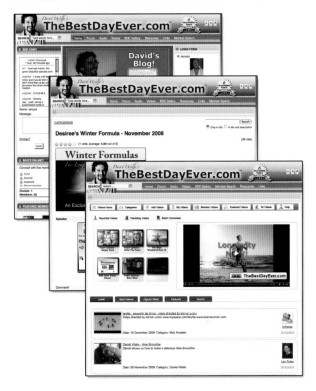

David Wolfe's Peak Performance Archives are available at www.thebestdayever.com.

Warning! The contents of this website may cause you to have The Best Day Ever!

This peak-performance website features a priceless amount of the most valuable information ever assembled in one place on peak performance and longevity, including nutritional seminars, documents, interviews, videos, product reviews, and product discounts for www.longevitywarehouse.com.

As soon as you join, you'll immediately have access to hundreds of MP3s, videos, PDFs, and much more. Even more importantly, inside www.thebestdayever.com is a community of individuals just like you. You can meet hundreds of new friends with the same passions for health, wellness, and success.

You'll learn how to:

- Shed those stubborn, unwanted pounds
- Achieve an extraordinary level of energy
- Utilize superfoods, superherbs, raw foods, and chocolate
- Discover up-to-date information from America's foremost healthy-lifestyle authorities
- Leap ahead of the curve in health, longevity, success technology, and peak performance
- Radically rejuvenate yourself physically, emotionally, and spiritually
- Enjoy every second of life, a second chance at life, and really experience The Best Day Ever
- Explode your creativity and imagination
- Sleep two to four fewer hours each night, and wake up feeling better than ever
- Add years (if not decades) to your life span

This incredible website gives you complete access to my text, audio, and video library, which contains hundreds of lectures and files on superfoods, superherbs, raw foods, chocolate, health, beauty, minerals, and rejuvenation programs, including information on how to heal some of the most stubborn ailments known to humanity. The website also includes professional nutrition coaching forums where you can get answers to your questions. You will hear live interviews with me on a monthly basis, where I answer your questions and bring you up to date on the latest and greatest news. Also, if you are interested, you can tap into my monthly blog on the site.

I am a strong believer in saturating oneself with positive, empowering information, so www.thebestdayever .com has been designed to bombard you with inspirational text, audio, and video.

All I do, all day, every day, is pursue and live the cutting edge of health, success, beauty, nutrition, longevity science, peak performance, and superfood/superherb diets. This information allows you to create astounding rejuvenation and healing *now,* without having to make the same mistakes that tens of thousands of others have made.

No more waiting by the mailbox. My website was created to give you immediate access to cutting-edge information that helps you instantly enhance the quality of your life. It is a constantly updated, ever-growing resource for you and your whole family to enjoy. This is the first time in the history of my career as a peak-performance consultant that I've grouped so many compelling, life-changing programs into one jam-packed website. Nothing else like this website is available on the Internet—it is truly a one-of-a-kind phenomenon.

If you are inspired to achieve an exceptional state of health, success, beauty, fitness, awareness, joy, sensuality, accomplishment, peak performance, and, most importantly, fun, then thebestdayever.com is for you!

JOIN TODAY and HAVE THE BEST DAY EVER!

Notes

Hail to the King! An Introduction to Chaga

1. N. Tzitzin et al., *Atlas of Medicinal Plants of the USSR* (in Russian, 1963).

2. Paul Stamets, *MycoMedicinals: An Informational Treatise on Mushrooms* (MycoMedia, 1999).

Part I: Facts and History of Use

1. Ron Spinosa, "The Chaga Story," *The Mycophile* 47, no. 1 (January/February 2006).

2. "Levitative" refers to the upward-tending force that provides a counterpart to gravity in a yin/yang type of relationship. In fact, the force of gravity cannot exist without the force of levity. If gravity were the only force or even the dominant one, then no growth could occur in our ecosystem. We would all be squashed flat, and that would be the end. Levity must actually be a greater force than gravity for growth to occur. A tree "falls" upward; it does not fight gravity, which would create heat, yet trees are cool. My observations have taught me that gravitational forces only exist (in the way we experience them) in the atmosphere, especially under the influence of light, heat, oxygen, and straight-line trajectories. Gravity can be shielded, blocked, or displaced. Levity occurs in the absence of light, heat, oxygen, and under the influence of double-spiral golden-mean (phi ratio) spiral patterns or pathways (such as tubules in bark), especially in high-hydrogen and Ormus mineral environments.

Newton asked the question: "Why did the apple fall from the tree?" A more insightful question would have been: "How did the apple get up there in the first place?"

3. www.survivaltopics.com/survival/the-chaga-natures-medicinal-mushroom.

4. Paul Stamets, *Mycelium Running: How Mushrooms Can Help Save the World* (Berkeley, CA: Ten Speed Press, 2005).

5. www.chagatrade.ru/betulin.html.

6. http://carner.ws/stories.

7. http://en.wikipedia.org/wiki/Shennong_Ben_Cao_Jing.

8. For more on the Santa Claus connection to *Amanita muscaria,* please visit the following three websites:

   http://aumstar.com/the-origin-of-saint-nikolaos-santa-claus-and-the-book-of-revelation

   www.cannabisculture.com/articles/3136.html

   www.atlanteanconspiracy.com/2008/09/santa-claus-magic-mushroom.html.

9. From www.aumstar.com. I presume that the mushroom growing in the immortal birch grove is chaga, but this website suggests that it is in fact *Amanita muscaria.* Interestingly, this website posits a version of the philosophical concept that the origin of the world's great languages unfolds from a hyperdimensional metaphysical information field contained in magic mushrooms of different types growing at the source of springs and headwaters of the world's greatest rivers.

9a. U. Peintner, R. Pöder, "Ethnomycological remarks on the Iceman's fungi," *The Iceman and his Natural Environment,* The Man in the Ice: Volume 4, 2000, pp 143–50.

Notes

9b. Both *Fomes fomentarius* and *Piptoporus betulinus* inhibit the growth of many problematic microorganisms including the bacteria: *P. aeruginosa* and *S. marcescens,* amongst others. *Piptoporus betulinus* also exhibits strong inhibitory activity against S. *aureus, B. subtilis,* and *M. smegmatis,* a cousin to the pathogenic Mycobacterium tuberculosis.

Paul Stamets, "Novel Antimicrobials from Mushrooms," *HerbalGram,* American Botanical Council, 2002; 54:28–33

10. This and all extracts from *The Cancer Ward,* by Aleksandr Solzhenitsyn, were taken from the September 1972 Bantam Books edition.

11. Chaga may be an exception to this rule, as it may be using melanin to produce energy, and melanin is known to chemically absorb the energy of solar radiation. This could explain why chaga produces exposed herniated mycelium (sclerotia), which would usually be inside the wood of the tree. Essentially, the chaga sclerotia emerges from the tree in order to capture sunlight and convert it into energy.

12. In a March 2011 personal communication with mycologist Paul Stamets, he stated that some mushrooms hyperaccumulate heavy metals, including radioactive debris such as cesium-137. For additional information, see Juan A. Campos, Noel A. Tejera, and Carlos J. Sánchez, "Substrate role in the accumulation of heavy metals in sporocarps of wild fungi," *Biometals* 22, no. 5 (October 2009): 835–41.

13. Murray Wittner and Louis Weiss, *The Microsporidia and Microsporidiosis* (Washington, DC: American Society for Microbiology, 1999), 199.

14. Terence McKenna, excerpt from the lecture "Tryptamine Hallucinogens and Consciousness," given at the Lilly-Goswami Conference on Consciousness and Quantum Physics at Esalen Institute (California) in December 1983. An edited transcription of this passage also appears in McKenna's book *The Archaic Revival* (New York: Harper San Francisco, 1991).

15. Martin Beech, "On Meteors and Mushrooms," *Journal of the Royal Astronomical Society of Canada* 81, no. 605 (April 1987), 27.

16. Francis Crick, *Life Itself: Its Origin and Nature* (New York: Simon and Schuster, 1981).

17. F. Hoyle, "Is the Universe Fundamentally Biological?" in *New Ideas in Astronomy,* eds. F. Bertola et al. (New York: Cambridge University Press, 1988), 5–8.

18. Lecture 5 of Botany 135, Fall 2003, University of Hawaii at Manoa, www.botany.hawaii.edu/faculty/wong/BOT35/Lect05_c.htm.

19. According to Bruce Moffett of the University of East London: "There is, they say, growing evidence that bacteria, fungal spores and viruses may spend large amounts of time—even their entire lives—in the air, riding clouds across the planet. And they don't just inhabit the clouds—they may also be creating them. Certainly, many of the clouds' newly discovered inhabitants are exquisitely designed to create the maximum number of ice crystals, the basic building-blocks of clouds.... The ecology of the atmosphere is one of the last great frontiers of biological exploration on Earth."

Until recently, scientists assumed that if the bacteria or fungi got caught up in the winds, they would be killed by ultraviolet radiation from the Sun. But Gene Shinn, of the U.S. Geological Survey in St. Petersburg, Florida, has examined their airborne lifestyle in detail. He says that the bacteria seem to protect themselves from harmful rays by becoming attached to dust particles. I will continue by quoting from http://brainmind.com/ScienceNews.html.

> In dust clouds, the amount of UV radiation will be lower than in "normal" situations. One of Shinn's USGS colleagues, Dale Griffin, suggests that bacteria might survive even longer if they get into cracks in the dust particles.
>
> Shinn has isolated more than 130 species of African bacteria and fungal spores over the Caribbean. Not only that, he says that they are probably responsible for a series of dramatic epidemics among Caribbean coral reefs in recent years.
>
> One example is an African soil fungus called *Aspergillus sydowii*. It was first spotted in the Caribbean in 1983 while Africa was affected by drought. Dust clouds blew into the upper atmosphere and traveled west on the trade winds, forming a dense haze over the waters of the Caribbean. Since those clouds brought *A. sydowii*, describes Shinn, the fungus has killed more than 90 percent of the region's soft coral sea fans.
>
> Many cloud-inhabiting and cloud-seeding bacteria design for themselves a protein that mimics the shape of an ice crystal's surface. This triggers the formation of ice crystals around which water vapor coalesces to create water droplets.
>
> Many bacteria seem to be able to form ice crystals, but the best equipped appears to be *Pseudomonas*

syringae, which commonly grows on plant matter, aiding the decomposition process. A single gram containing a million bacteria could theoretically produce up to a million ice crystals. It can trigger the formation of ice at temperatures of 13°C, higher than other "ice nucleators." This ability is so well known that the bacteria are sometimes added to the water put into snow-making machines at ski resorts. In the atmosphere, the bacteria create clouds. *Pseudomonas syringae* has been found in the core of hailstones.

20. In research sponsored by the Dove Health Alliance and performed by Brunswick Labs (dated September 27, 2005), an alcohol extract of wild Siberian chaga tested at 52,452 micromoles TE per liter. This ORAC measurement indicates a high antioxidant content. For a comparison to other mushrooms, maitake tested at 15,977, cordyceps at 12,328, reishi at 4,934, and agaricus at 1,298 (micromoles TE per liter). Please consider (in terms of comparing to other data) that these units are "per liter," not "per gram."

20a.http://www.readcube.com/articles/10.1038/ja.2011.2

21. http://carner.ws/stories.

22. Ibid. And a reminder: Chaga grows in the entire cir-cumpolar region of the northern hemisphere of the Earth, not only Siberia.

23. www.bioportfolio.com/resources/pmarticle/160347 /Rapid-Isolation-And-Purification-Of-Inotodiol-And-Trametenolic-Acid-From-Inonotus-Obliquus.html.

24. http://en.wikipedia.org/wiki/Ergosterol.

25. David Wolfe and Dr. Joseph Mercola, *The Healing Power of Vitamin D*, booklet (Los Angeles: New Horizon Health, 2009).

26. Ibid.

27. www.webmd.com/multiple-sclerosis/news/20090428
/high-doses-vitamin-d-cut-ms-relapses.
28. http://jcem.endojournals.org/content/89/11/5387.full.
29. www.earthbornwellness.com/chagause.htm.
30. Ibid.
31. http://carner.ws/stories.
32. K. Kahlos, L. Kangas, and R. Hiltunen, "Antitumor activity of some compounds and fractions from an n-hexane extract of *Inonotus obliquus* in vitro," *Acta Pharm Fennica* 96 (1987): 33–40.
33. M. Nomura et al., "Inotodiol, a Lanostane Triterpenoid, from *Inonotus obliquus* Inhibits Cell Proliferation through Caspase-3-dependent Apoptosis," *Anticancer Research* 28 (2008): 2691–96.
34. Xiu-hong Zhong, Li-bo Wang, and Dong-zhi Sun, "Effects of inotodiol extracts from inonotus obliquus on proliferation cycle and apoptotic gene of human lung adenocarcinoma cell line A549," *Chinese Journal of Integrative Medicine* 17, no. 3 (2011): 218–23.
35. Mi Ja Chung, Cha-Kwon Chung, Yoonhwa Jeong, and Seung-Shi Ham, "Anticancer activity of subfractions containing pure compounds of Chaga mushroom (Inonotus obliquus) extract in human cancer cells and in Balbc/c mice bearing Sarcoma-180 cells," *Nutr Res Pract.*, 4, no. 3 (June 2010): 177–82.
36. Yeon-Ran Kim, "Immunomodulatory Activity of the Water Extract from Medicinal Mushroom *Inonotus obliquus*," *Mycobiology* 33, no. 3 (September 2005): 158–62.

Abstract from this study: The immunomodulatory effect of aqueous extract of *Inonotus obliquus*, called Chaga, was tested on bone marrow cells from chemically immunosuppressed mice. The Chaga water extract was daily administered for 24 days to mice that had been treated with cyclophosphamide (400 mg/kg body weight), immunosuppressive alkylating agent. The number of colony-forming unit (CFU)-granulocytes/macrophages (GM) and erythroid burst-forming unit (BFU-E) increased almost to the levels seen in non-treated control as early as 8 days after treatment. Oral administration of the extract highly increased serum levels of IL-6. Also, the level of TNF-α was elevated by the chemical treatment in control mice, whereas was maintained at the background level in the extract-treated mice, indicating that the extract might effectively suppress TNF- related pathologic conditions. These results strongly suggest the great potential of the aqueous extract from Inonotus obliquus as immune enhancer during chemotherapy.

See also: I. M. Thompson, C. R. Spence, D. L. Lamm, and N. R. DiLuzio (November 1987), "Immunochemotherapy of bladder carcinoma with glucan and cyclophosphamide," *The American Journal of the Medical Sciences* (United States: Lippincott Williams & Wilkins) 294, no. 5: 294–300.

A. Wakui et al., "Randomized study of lentinan on patients with advanced gastric and colorectal cancer. Tohoku Lentinan Study Group" [in Japanese]. *Cancer & Chemotherapy* (Japanese: *Gan To Kagaku Ryohosha* 13, no. 4-1 (April 1986): 1050–59.

37. M. L. Patchen, M. M. D'Alesandro, I. Brook, W. F. Blakely, T. J. McVittie, "Glucan: Mechanisms Involved in Its 'Radioprotective' Effect," *Journal of Leukocyte Biology* 42 (1987): 95–105.

38. D. Akramiene, A. Kondrotas, J. Didziapetriene, E. Kevelaitis, "Effects of Beta-Glucans on the Immune System," *Medicina (Kaunas)* 43, no. 8 (2007): 597–606.

    See also: Daniel E. Cramer et al., "Beta-Glucan Enhances Complement-Mediated Hematopoietic Recovery after Bone Marrow Injury," *Blood* 107, no. 2 (2006): 835–40.

39. A. A. Tohamy et al., "Beta-Glucan Inhibits the Genotoxicity of Cyclophosphamide, Adriamycin and Cisplatin," *Mutation Research* 541, nos. 1 and 2 (November 2003): 45–53.

40. G. Sener, E. Eksioglu-Demiraop, M. Cetiner, F. Ercan, B. C. Yegen, "Beta-Glucan Ameliorates Methotrexate-Induced Oxidative Organ Injury via Its Antioxidant and Immunomodulatory Effects," *European Journal of Pharmacology* 542, nos. 1–3 (2006): 170–78.

41. Sudhakar Chintharlapalli, Sabitha Papineni, Shashi K. Ramaiah, and Stephen Safe, "Betulinic Acid Inhibits Prostate Cancer Growth through Inhibition of Specificity Protein Transcription Factors," *Cancer Research* 67, no. 6 (2007): 2816–23.

42. Bokyung Sung et al., "Identification of a Novel Blocker of I B Kinase Activation That Enhances Apoptosis and Inhibits Proliferation and Invasion by Suppressing Nuclear Factor-B," *Molecular Cancer Therapeutics* 7, no. 1 (2008): 191–201.

43. According to Russia's Saratov State University, 1932.

44. Medical Encyclopedia (Moscow, 1965).

Part II: Preparing and Enjoying Chaga

 1. Sook Jong Rhee et al., "A comparative study of analytical methods for alkali-soluble β-glucan in medicinal

mushroom, Chaga *(Inonotus obliquus)*" *LWT—Food Science and Technology* 41, no. 3 (April 2008): 545–49.

2. Ron Spinosa (January/February 2006), "The Chaga Story," *The Mycophile* 47, no. 1.

3. For more about this program, go to www.longevity nowprogram.com and click on "Longevity Now Program."

4. Paul Kouchakoff's research is often referenced by raw-food advocates. Kouchakoff essentially overturned the previously held idea that eating any kind of food causes leukocytosis and immune system activation. Kouchakoff demonstrated that eating cooking food above a certain critical temperature causes leukocytosis. He showed that heating water above (191°F or 88°C) and then drinking that water (when cooled down) causes leukocytosis, whereas below that temperature it does not. Repeated leukocytosis due to drinking boiled water or eating cooked food is essentially an excessive stress on the immune system. These details are found in the proceedings of the first international Congress of Microbiology (Paris 1930): "The Influence of Cooking on the Blood Formula of Man" by Paul Kouchakoff, MD, of the Institute of Clinical Chemistry, Lausanne, Switzerland. (Translation by Lee Foundation for Nutritional Research, Milwaukee, Wisconsin.)

Part III: The Science on Chaga

The following website can be used as a resource for all the scientific material touched upon in this section: www.chagatrade.ru/betulin.html.

Notes

1. Margaret M. O'Connell, Michael D. Bentleya, Christopher S. Campbell, and Barbara J. W. Colea, "Betulin and Lupeol in Bark from Four White-Barked Birches," *Phytochemistry* 27, no. 7 (1988): 2175–76.

2. See also A. Felföldi-Gáva et al., "Betulaceae and Platanaceae Plants as Alternative Sources of Selected Lupane-Type Triterpenes: Their Composition Profile and Betulin Content," *Journal Acta Chromatographica* 21, no. 4 (Akadémiai Kiadó, December 2009): 671–81.

3. See www.betterhealththruresearch.com/340Research PapersChaga.htm, www.chagamushroom.com/chaga _researcher_endorsements.htm, and www.earthborn -wellness.com/chagause.htm.

4. http://ralphmoss.com/html/betu.shtml.

5. Sebastian Jäger, Melanie N. Laszczyk, and Armin Scheffler, "A Preliminary Pharmacokinetic Study of Betulin, the Main Pentacyclic Triterpene from Extract of Outer Bark of Birch (Betulae alba cortex)," *Molecules* 13, no. 12 (December 2008): 3224–35.

6. Paul Stamets, *Mycelium Running: How Mushrooms Can Help Save the World* (Berkeley, CA: Ten Speed Press, 2005). Referencing K. Kahlos, L. Kangas, and R. Hiltunen, "Antitumor activity of some compounds and fractions from an n-hexane extract of *Inonotus obliquus* in vitro," *Acta Pharm Fennica* 96 (1987): 33–40.

7. Jan H. Kessler, Franziska B. Mullauer, Guido M. de Roo, and Jan Paul Medema, "Broad In Vitro Efficacy of Plant-Derived Betulinic Acid against Cell Lines Derived from the Most Prevalent Human Cancer Types," *Cancer Letters* 251, no. 1 (June 2007): 132–45.

8. M. S. de Sá, J. F. Costa, A. U. Krettli, M. G. Zalis, G.

L. Maia, I. M. Sette, A. Câmara Cde, J. M. Filho, A. M. Giulietti-Harley, R. Ribeiro Dos Santos, and M. B. Soares (July 2009), "Antimalarial activity of betulinic acid and derivatives in vitro against *Plasmodium falciparum* and in vivo in *P. berghei*-infected mice." *Parasitol Res.* 105, no. 1: 275–89.

9. Valentina Zuco et al., "Selective Cytotoxicity of Betulinic Acid on Tumor Cell Lines, but Not on Normal Cells," *Cancer Letters* 175, no. 1 (January 2002): 17–25.

10. Young Geun Shin et al., "Determination of Betulinic Acid in Mouse Blood, Tumor and Tissue Homogenates by Liquid Chromatography–Electrospray Mass Spectrometry," *Journal of Chromatography B: Biomedical Sciences and Applications* 732, no. 2 (September 1999): 331–36.

11. See U.S. Patent 5750578: Use of Betulin and Analogs Thereof to Treat Herpes Virus Infection.

12. Yunha Yun et al., "Immunomodulatory Activity of Betulinic Acid by Producing Pro-Inflammatory Cytokines and Activation of Macrophages," *Archives of Pharmacal Research* 26, no. 12 (2003): 1087–95.

13. www.chagatrade.ru/betulin.html.

14. S. P. Wasser, "Medicinal mushrooms as a source of antitumor and immunomodulating polysaccharides," *Appl Microbiol Biotechnol.* 60, no. 3 (November 2002): 258–74.

15. B. C. Lehtovaara and F. X. Gu, "Pharmacological, Structural, and Drug Delivery Properties and Applications of 1,3-ß-Glucans," *Journal of Agricultural and Food Chemistry* 59, no. 13 (June 2011): 6813–28.

   See also: G. Kogan et al., "Yeast Cell Wall Polysaccharides as Antioxidants and Antimutagens: Can They Fight Cancer?" *Neoplasma* 55, no. 5 (2008): 387–93.

M. Rondanelli, A. Opizzi, F. Monteferrario, "The Biological Activity of Beta-Glucans," *Minerva Medical* 100, no. 3 (June 2009): 237–45.

16. Susanta Banik, "Mushrooms: The Magic Store of Health Benefits," *Everyman's Science* XLIV, no. 6 (February/March 2010): 360–65.

See also: D. Akramiene, A. Kondrotas, J. Didziape-triene, and E. Kevelaitis, "Effects of Beta-Glucans on the Immune System," *Medicina (Kaunas)* 43, no. 8 (2007): 597–606.

Yoo Kyoung Park et al., "Chaga Mushroom Extract Inhibits Oxidative DNA Damage in Human Lympho-cytes as Assessed by Comet Assay," *Biofactors* 21, nos. 1–4 (2004): 109–12.

Yana Song et al., "Identification of *Inonotus obliquus* (Chaga) and Analysis of Antioxidation and Antitumor Activities of Polysaccharides," *Current Microbiology* 57, no. 5 (2008): 454–62.

Sung Hak Lee et al., "Antitumor Activity of Water Ex-tract of a Mushroom, *Inonotus obliquus,* against HT-29 Human Colon Cancer Cells," *Phytotherapy Research* 23, no. 12 (December 2009): 1784–89.

Seung-Shi Hama et al., "Antimutagenic Effects of Subfractions of Chaga Mushroom *(Inonotus obliquus)* Extract," *Mutation Research* 672 (2009): 55–59.

17. M. L. Patchen and T. J. MacVittie, "Temporal Response of Murine Pluripotent Stem Cells and Myeloid and Erythroid Progenitor Cells to Low-Dose Glucan Treat-ment," *Acta Haematologica* 70, no. 5 (1983): 281–88.

18. M. L. Patchen et al. (1984), "Proliferation of Stem Cells, Promoting White Blood Cell Recovery in Bone Marrow Injury and Repair," *J. Biol. Res. Mod.* 3: 627–33.

19. G. C. Chan, W. K. Chan, and D. M. Sze, "The Effects of Beta-Glucan on Human Immune and Cancer Cells," *Journal of Hematology and Oncology* 2 (June 10, 2009): 25.

20. Joyce K. Czop, "The Role of Beta Glucan Receptors on Blood and Tissue Leukocytes in Phagocytosis and Metabolic Activation," *Pathology and Immunopathology Research* 5 (1986): 286–96.

21. Stephen J. Delatte, Jill Evans, Andre Hebra, William Adamson, H. Biemann Othersen, and Edward P. Tagge, "Effectiveness of beta-glucan collagen for treatment of partial-thickness burns in children," *Journal of Pediatric Surgery* 36, no. 1 (January 2001): 113–18.

22. M. L. Patchen, M. M. D'Alesandro, I. Brook, W. F. Blakely, and T. J. MacVittie, "Glucan: mechanisms involved in its 'radioprotective' effect," *J. Leukoc. Biol.* 42, no. 2 (August 1987): 95–105.

23. Leonid Ber, "Beta-1,3-D-Glucan: The Skin Connection," *Nature's Impact* (December 1997).

24. H. Z. Toklu and G. Sener, "Beta-Glucan Protects against Burn-Induced Oxidative Organ Damage in Rats," *International Immunopharmacology* 6, no. 2 (2006): 156–69.

25. E. A. Dosychev and V. N. Bystrova, "Treatment of Psoriasis with Chaga," *Vestnik Dermatologii i Venerologii* 47, no. 5 (May 1973): 79–83.

26. Valentina G. Babitskaya et al., "Melanin Complex of Medicinal Mushroom *Inonotus Obliquus*," *International Journal of Medical Mushrooms* 4 (2002): 139–45.

27. M. L. Barrenäs and F. Lindgren, "The Influence of Inner Ear Melanin on Susceptibility to TTS in Humans," *Scandinavian Audiology,* 19, no. 2 (1990): 97–102.

28. David Wilcock, *The Source Field Investigations* (New York: Dutton [Penguin], 2011).

29. Chaga is my #1 superherb recommendation for those with vitiligo.

29a. Dadachova E, Bryan RA, Huang X, Moadel T, Schweitzer AD, Aisen P, Nosanchuk JD, Casadevall A. (2007). Rutherford, Julian, ed. "Ionizing radiation changes the electronic properties of melanin and enhances the growth of melanized fungi". PLoS ONE 2 (5): e457. doi:10.1371/journal.pone.0000457. PMC 1866175. PMID 17520016.

30. Pierre Beaumier, PhD, CChem, Fellow of the Chemical Institute of Canada and president of CanAlt Health Labs. Ramiz Saad, BSc, President of Triangle of Life Products, Inc.

31. *International Journal of Medicinal Mushrooms* 13, no. 2 (2011): 121–30.

32. *American Journal of Pharmacology and Toxicology* 2 (2007): 10–17.

33. *International Journal of Medicinal Mushrooms* 13, no. 2 (2011): 121–30.

34. *Chemical and Pharmaceutical Bulletin* 55, no. 8 (2007): 1222–26.

35. Lewis J. Moorman, "Health of the Navajo–Hopi Indians," *JAMA* 139, no. 6 (February 5, 1949).

36. Centers for Disease Control and National Institutes of Health, Health People 2010, "3: Cancer," www.health.gov/healthpeople/document/HTML/Volume1/03Cancer.htm.

37. *Food Additives and Contaminants* 25 (2008): 51–58.
38. *Journal of Environmental Radioactivity* 102 (2000): 386–92.
39. *Pharmacology, Biochemistry, and Behaviour* 21 (1984): 1–5.
40. *Pharmacology, Biochemistry, and Behaviour* 21, supplement 1 (1984): 3–11.

Index

About the Author

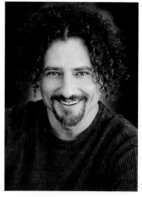

Photo by Michael Roud

David "Avocado" Wolfe (born August 6, near New York City) is considered by peers to be one of the world's leading authorities on nutrition. David develops and distributes some of the planet's most wonderful and exotic organic food items. David was the first to bring raw and organic cacao beans/nibs (raw chocolate), goji berries, Incan berries, cacao butter, cacao powder, powdered encapsulated mangosteen, maca extract, cold-pressed coconut oil, and Sacred Chocolate™ into general distribution in North America. Known for extraordinary quality control and ethical production, these products and many others developed by David lead the field.

David brings a unique perspective on health and nutrition to the world of superherbs and superfoods. He holds degrees in mechanical and environmental engineering, political science, a Juris doctor in law degree, and a master's degree in living-food nutrition. He has studied at many institutions, including Oxford University. Since 1995, David has hosted over 2,700 health lectures, conferences, educational dinners, and seminars in North America, Central America, South

America, Africa, the Middle East, Oceania, Asia, and Australia. As part of his action-packed schedule, David also coaches and feeds Hollywood producers and celebrities, as well as some of the world's leading business people and entrepreneurs. The author of *Superfoods, The Sunfood Diet Success System, Naked Chocolate, Eating for Beauty,* and *Amazing Grace,* he also hosts health, fitness, and adventure retreats each year at various sites around the world. You may view his current schedule at www.davidwolfe.com.

David is the founder of and chief contributor to the Internet's leading peak-performance and nutrition magazine: www.thebestdayever.com. He is also founder of the nonprofit Fruit Tree Planting Foundation (www .ftpf.org), whose goal is to plant eighteen billion fruit trees on planet Earth. David's products are available via www.longevitywarehouse.com and health-food stores internationally.

Other than his passion for nutrition, David's favorite hobbies include drumming, gardening, hiking, yoga, literature, writing, alchemy, chemistry, wild adventures, hot-springs soaking, planting fruit trees, spending time with loved ones, and having The Best Day Ever!

Main website:
davidwolfe.com

Shop:

longevitywarehouse.com

sacredchocolate.com

Learn:

thebestdayever.com

longevityconference.com

womenswellnessconference.com

rawnutritioncertification.com

Travel:

davidwolfeadventures.com

Non-profit:

ftpf.org

Connect:

twitter.com/DavidWolfe

facebook.com/DavidAvocadoWolfe

youtube.com/DavidAvocadoWolfe

instagram.com/DavidAvocadoWolfe

To book David Wolfe on a television or radio show, for an interview, or for a seminar, please contact Angela Hartman at angela@ahartmaninc.com.

"The subtle energy of your food becomes your mind."

— Upanishads

The Fruit Tree Planting Foundation

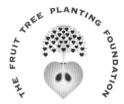

www.ftpf.org

"Nothing in the world gives me more satisfaction than planting fruit, nut, and medicinal trees. As I have always chosen to channel my energy and finances into environmentally friendly, sustainable, and healthy directions, I founded the nonprofit Fruit Tree Planting Foundation so that we can all vote with our money for a better, happier, more abundant, forested future on Earth. Please read about our foundation and decide that you want to donate your time, energy and/or finances to this worthy cause."

—DAVID WOLFE

The Fruit Tree Planting Foundation (FTPF) is a unique nonprofit charity dedicated to planting edible, fruitful trees and plants to benefit needy populations and improve the surrounding air, soil, and water. We strategically plant orchards where the harvest will best serve the local community for decades to follow, at places such as Native American reservations, city parks, homeless shelters, drug rehab centers, low-income areas, international hunger relief sites, and animal sanctuaries. FTPF's projects benefit the environment, human health, and animal welfare—all at once!

FTPF's goal is straightforward: to collectively plant eighteen billion fruit, nut, and medicinal trees for a healthy planet (approximately three for every person alive).

Fruit, nut, and medicinal trees heal the environment by cleaning the air, improving soil quality, preventing erosion, creating animal habitats, sustaining valuable water sources, and providing healthy nutrition. We envision a place where one can have a summer picnic under the shade of a fruit, nut, or medicinal tree, breathe the clean air it generates, listen to the songbirds it attracts, and not have to bring anything other than an appetite for the healthy foods growing overhead.

We envision and act to create a world where one can take a walk in the park during a lunch break, pick and eat a variety of delicious fruits, plant the seeds so others can eventually do the same, and provide an alternative to buying environmentally destructive, illness-causing, chemically laden products. FTPF has planted hundreds of thousands of fruit trees all over the world and provided advice and training for others to do the same. We have launched a series of exciting new programs, and we need your help! Your tax-deductible, charitable investment will help us realize our dream of a sustainable planet for generations to come. As you find you are interested in donating, please send a check or money order payable to:

The Fruit Tree Planting Foundation

The Fruit Tree Planting Foundation
P.O. Box 81881
Pittsburgh, PA 15217

Donations may also be made online at
www.ftpf.org

or by contacting the foundation by phone or email:

info@ftpf.org
Telephone: 831-621-8096
Toll-free: 877-884-7570
Fax: 831-621-7978

We will send a receipt for your tax-deductible dona-
tion, but you may also want to make a note of this trans-
action for tax purposes. Thank you for taking action.

Final Words

Herbalism fosters ecological literacy. The deeper you go into herbal lore and wisdom, the deeper you go into an environmentally friendly and sustainable lifestyle. Herbalism teaches us that the great herbs of the world are an open treasure to us all, especially in every evolved ecosystem. Supporting healthy, natural, original ecosystems allows us to access the greater, more potent herbs for healing and expanding consciousness. And in already disturbed ecosystems (suburbs, cities, abandoned industrial land, etc.), herbalism is an ecological force for good as it offers the intent and ability to identify, plant, and nourish the great herbs that inevitably create a healthy and health-giving landscape.

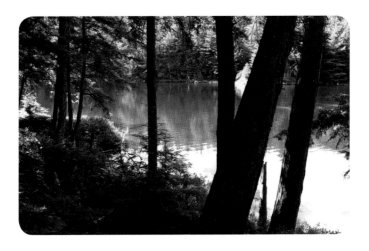